Crisis Intervention
in the Schools

The Guilford School Practitioner Series

EDITORS

STEPHEN N. ELLIOTT, Ph.D.
University of Wisconsin—Madison

JOSEPH C. WITT, Ph.D.
Louisiana State University, Baton Rouge

CRISIS INTERVENTION IN THE SCHOOLS

GAYLE D. PITCHER, Ph.D.
SCOTT POLAND, Ed.D.

THE GUILFORD PRESS
New York   London

© 1992 The Guilford Press
A Division of Guilford Publications, Inc.
72 Spring Street, New York, NY 10012

Printed in the United States of America

This book is printed on acid-free paper.

Last digit is print number: 9   8   7   6   5

Library of Congress Cataloging-in-Publication Data

Pitcher, Gayle Diane.
    Crisis intervention in the schools / Gayle D. Pitcher and Scott Poland.
        p.   cm. — (The Guilford school practitioner series)
    Includes bibliographical references and index.
    ISBN 0-89862-243-3.   ISBN 0-89862-364-2
    1. School psychology—United States.   2. Crisis intervention (Psychiatry)—United States.   3. School children—United States—Mental health services.   4. High school students—United States—Mental health services.   I. Poland, Scott. II. Title.
III. Series.
    [DNLM: 1. Counseling. 2. Crisis Intervention. 3. Mental Health Services. 4. School Health Services. WA 352 P682c]
LB1027.55.P53   1992
371.7—dc20
DNLM/DLC
for Library of Congress   92-1417
                                            CIP

Preface

President Bush and the governors of all 50 states recently set the goal that by the year 2000 every school in America would be free of drugs and violence. Crisis incidents in the schools of this country appear to be at an all-time high. The following newspaper headlines illustrate the complexity and severity of the crisis events that occur in the schools:

- Four skip school killed in crash (1987, December 5). *Houston Post,* p. A-1.
- Student takes official hostage (1987, December 8). *Houston Post,* p. A-1.
- Car hits elemtnary school; 2 die (1988, April 29). *Houston Post,* p. A-17.
- Twelve employees treated after chemical spill at school (1987, June 24). *Tulsa Tribune,* p. A-12.
- Tennessee teacher charged in death of assistant principal, fire (1990, May 22). *USA Today,* p. A-3.
- Boy hits head, dies in gym accident (1987, June 14). *Houston Post,* p. C-3.
- Six killed in traffic accident: School bus, tractor trailer collide in Florida (1987, August 29). *Houston Post,* p. A-12.
- U.S.A. schools wrestle with kid violence (1989, February 2). *USA Today,* p. A-1.
- Students urged to talk about Arkansas killings (1988, January 5) *Houston Post,* p. E-4.
- Schools disturbed by rowdy fans (1987, September 30). *USA Today,* p. D-1.
- Spate of school shootings continue in weeks after California slayings (1989, February 5). *Education Week,* p. 6.

- Gun toting teacher settles rowdy students (1990, March 27). *Houston Chronicle,* p. A-3.
- Former educational gem struggles with violence (1990, April 24). *Houston Chronicle,* p. A-3.

Few schools are prepared to face such severe crisis events. Crisis intervention has not been a part of the preparation for any group of school professionals. We personally experienced such severe crisis situations in our district as students and faculty being shot and numerous student suicides. We were unprepared to face such tragic situations, although we did the best that we could under the circumstances. Schools have been slow to develop crisis plans and have devoted few resources to the most important area of crisis intervention, which is, How can we prevent a crisis from occurring?

There is a growing awareness of the need for better crisis planning in the schools. School administrators will undoubtedly be held more accountable for crisis planning in the near future. Recent national headlines have brought to everyone's attention the amount of crime and violence that occurs on college campuses. National legislation requires that colleges now report campus crimes. It is hoped that similar legislation will be enacted for elementary and secondary schools. Everyone wants children to attend a safe school, but to ensure that will require much effort. Our schools will need to make safety a priority, and community agencies and parents will have to be involved. This book is written to provide a theoretical basis of crisis intervention and practical examples.

We are very appreciative of the support that we have received from the administrators in the Cypress-Fairbanks Independent School District. Our administrators have made crisis intervention a priority.

Contents

1

Introduction

WHY CRISIS INTERVENTION?

We have been working as psychologists in the schools for nearly 10 years. Prior to that we had received traditional training in education and psychology, including assessment of children and adolescents, consultation, family and individual therapy, learning theory, and psychopathology. My (Dr. Pitcher) internship and postdoctoral work were in a clinical setting, so my preparation included both educational and clinical aspects. During my training, I worked evenings and weekends in the psychiatric emergency room of a major urban medical center, Parkland Hospital, under Douglas Puryear (1979, author of *Helping People in Crisis*). The cases we saw there were the most severe and chronic psychopathology in crisis: mental illness warrants, family violence, substance abuse, violent and psychotic adults. Scott (Dr. Poland) also spent years working in inpatient facilities for psychiatrically disabled individuals.

"Everyday" Crises in the Schools

On accepting employment with a school district, we were prepared to focus on aspects of basically healthy children: to enhance their learning, to support self-esteem, and to help teachers manage mild behavior problems. We were wrong. The cases we consistently found ourselves involved with were as severe as those moving through the psychiatric emergency room and community mental health system, albeit at a younger age. In education, however, we are asked to manage severe cases with fewer resources; we cannot ask our on-site medical director to

1

order sedatives, and we cannot call the orderly when someone becomes physically aggressive.

We would have been awe-stricken had we been told during our training of what lay ahead, that we would be working with students who had spent time in the state correctional institution; that my nose would be broken by an angry adolescent; that we would be called to participate in crisis intervention following violent attacks on teachers; and that suicide intervention, child abuse, working with students upset by death and divorce, and commitment procedures would be regular features of our week. We did not expect that the training and experience that we had gained in the Parkland Hospital psychiatric emergency room or in state inpatient psychiatric facilities would often be applicable and even indispensable training for working in a school district. It was.

Why aren't severe child psychiatric disorders or crises attended to in community, clinical, or even residential mental health settings? Common reasons we have encountered usually fall into four general categories:

1. The child/adolescent or the family does not recognize the need for mental health services.
2. The child and the family are so dysfunctional they cannot organize involvement with community agencies.
3. No low-cost or affordable alternatives are available within reasonable distance.
4. For one reason or another the child and family have "burned their bridges" with other local mental health agencies.

It is not difficult to see that the above group of individuals who are in crisis and need services in the school setting are often the most severe group in terms of general psychological/emotional functioning. Further, recent trends in mental health and society at large have moved the crisis intervention arena more and more into the community: divorce, crime, and drug abuse are on the rise; disturbed children and adolescents are released from state inpatient facilities in record time; private facilities are almost never affordable as a long-term solution; and treatment philosophy moves more and more in the direction of community-based, least-restrictive (and -expensive) alternatives.

School personnel are asked more and more to intervene with serious emotional and developmental crises because there is usually no alternative. The school is the only community institution where all children come together every day, and school staffs provide expertise in dispensing guidance. Further, schools have a great stake in resolving these problems: Children who are in emotional or physical pain do not learn well.

Where do troubled children and adolescents go when released from residential facilities? To the public schools. Where do juvenile delinquents go when they return from an institutional setting? Very often they are enrolled in school. When state hospitals empty their back wards and prisons release adults aged 21 or younger, these populations have the option of returning to school. Since implementation of PL 94-142, the public schools must offer these individuals an appropriate program. Although many "at-risk" students function appropriately when they are placed in a supportive educational setting, many do not. The chance for crisis increases.

The Role of the School Psychologist in Crisis Intervention

The school environment has changed quite substantially in the past few decades. This trend is illustrated dramatically in the comparison between the top discipline problems in rural Canadian schools between the 1940s and the 1980s (Fullerton Police Department, 1987). Times have clearly changed.

1940s	*1980s*
1. Talking	1. Drug and alcohol abuse
2. Chewing gum	2. Pregnancy
3. Making noise	3. Suicide
4. Running in the halls	4. Rape
5. Getting out of turn in line	5. Robbery, burglary, assault
6. Wearing improper clothing	6. Arson, bombings
7. Not putting paper in wastebaskets	7. Murder
	8. Absenteeism
	9. Vandalism
	10. Extortion
	11. Gang warfare
	12. Abortion
	13. Venereal disease

Crisis intervention may not have been a significant need 50 years ago, but at present it clearly is. The need for crisis intervention skills to be included in the training and job descriptions of school personnel such as administrators, counselors, and school psychologists is being cited more frequently as an essential to keep our schools safe and emotionally healthy (Guetzloe, 1988; Nelson & Slaikeu, 1984; Sandoval, 1985). Stevens (1990, p. 2) comments:

In the snow-covered High Sierra Mountains of Lake Tahoe it is said that there are two kinds of drivers: those who have driven into a snowbank and those who are about to. Similarly, there are two types of school administrators: those who have faced a major crisis and those who are about to.

Despite Stevens's warnings that school districts avoid "getting caught with their (crisis) plans down" few schools to date have developed crisis intervention plans in any comprehensive way.

What's more, few programs in psychology or education include such training. A degree in mental health—as counselor, psychologist, psychiatrist, social worker—does not necessarily imply knowledge of crisis intervention. Many mental health professionals working in the schools have not received any training in crisis intervention. Although few of us may feel completely prepared to face and manage the barrage of crises that occur among children and adolescents, the simple reality is that most of us will, even those of us in "successful" schools and prominent neighborhoods (Jay, 1989). National statistics on school-related crises bear out this observation and are summarized in the following section.

Apparently our work in the schools—primarily consultation, direct counseling services, and crisis intervention—is not characteristic of that of the typical school psychologist. Crisis intervention appears to be in its infancy in the school setting. Although most school psychologists rate the need or desire for crisis intervention activities highly, they spend the major portion of their time with assessment activities apparently because of special education funding restrictions (Carroll, Harris, & Bretzing, 1979; Cook & Patterson, 1977; Lacayo, Sherwood, & Morris, 1981).

Although ongoing debates regarding the propriety of long-term counseling or psychotherapy in schools rage on (Sandoval, 1985), crisis needs surface frequently in classrooms. These demand immediate attention and cannot be ignored—a child throws a chair across his classroom, an adolescent girl breaks down in tears during an English literature class, a young man claims he is going home to kill himself, a school bus accident results in several student deaths. As we discuss in forthcoming chapters, one of the absolute necessities of crisis intervention is immediacy. A child, adolescent, or school in crisis needs immediate attention in order to restore normal emotional functioning or at least to stabilize emotional functioning. This strategy appeals to basic, human common sense; when we see someone who is too acutely upset to function in school, our basic instincts tell us to do something to ease the pain.

These individuals need emotional first aid immediately, and, in day-to-day practice, caring human beings make their best attempt to support them; this support roster includes secretaries, bus drivers, teachers, parent volunteers, counselors, principals, and school psychologists. A formal referral to the community, on the other hand, may result in weeks on a waiting list and, for various reasons, is all too frequently not followed through by the family. Since this sort of home-spun emotional first aid typically is delivered without training, it probably would benefit all school personnel to receive some basic, practical skill training in providing support to children and adolescents in emotional duress.

It seems logical and appropriate that psychologists working in the schools take primary responsibility for such training. Although other mental health professionals in the schools might also fill this role, it is most important that it be addressed. Further, school psychologists write again and again about expanding the assessment role to include direct services to regular education students and to wed direct services with a broader range of preventive mental health activities (Sandoval, 1986). Crisis counseling and crisis intervention mesh well with this model, and it is likely that such a role will be heartily welcomed by other school personnel. Principals and counselors appreciate quick, efficient help in times of crisis, are exasperated when the school psychologist cannot be reached during a crisis, and frequently seek out the psychologist when he or she is not in the building (Sandoval, 1985).

It is a challenge to recognize that crises will occur. Subsequent to each crisis we breathe a sigh of relief with the impression that it was a very extraordinary occurrence that we will, thank goodness, never again encounter. We cling to our training and early impressions that we should be working with less severe problems in schools or that we really need to focus only on education despite continuing evidence to the contrary.

Crisis in Groups: Building Crises and Disasters

Working directly with individual students and staff members in crisis was the most immediate and regular aspect of our crisis functioning in the schools. A few years after our department began operation, however, we came face to face with a whole new horizon of crisis intervention—crises that affected whole buildings, districts, and even communities.

No one on our staff will forget the first major incident we were involved in. Psychological services received a desperate call from a high school just after a student, dressed in camouflage, had gunned down a principal and a fellow student in a crowded cafeteria. As professional psychologists we were expected to contribute significantly to the amelioration of the situation. Our anxiety levels soared, and the temptation to avoid the situation altogether was strong. The truth was that we knew little more than the average layperson about intervening in organizational disaster. This awareness produced the same tension and "disequilibrium" for us as for those directly involved in the disaster.

What we found at the school confirmed our worst expectations. Television news teams roamed the halls, large numbers of frightened students were unaccounted for, telephone lines were clogged with frantic calls from parents, teachers were rattled from the near hysteria and uncertainty. Understandably, administrators felt ill-equipped to manage the barrage of problems that had fallen on them in the course of a fleeting moment.

Even though these organizational crises occur infrequently, in the course of a professional lifetime, they occur with predictable regularity. We can anticipate and prepare for them just as we do for fires. School districts that get caught with their "plans down" may have a great deal of difficulty facing the community. In our experience a major organizational crisis should be expected (in a moderate-sized to large school district) almost every year. In the years we have been working in our 41,00-enrollment Texas district we have encountered one sniper assault, one shooting of a principal in school, several suicides that affected large numbers of the student population, a case of threatened violence to children through telephone calls, a food poisoning scare, and numerous deaths of students and staff as a result of illness, accidents, or murder. Since school psychologists and mental health workers in general deal with individuals in crisis, and since they are often more transient and able to cancel appointments, it is logical that they be involved with management of these organizational crises and probably instrumental in developing an ongoing plan for their continuing management.

Plan of the Book

This book is intended to be a practical handbook for individuals working in the schools. Whatever the reason, it is clear that crises are no longer unique events that will rarely or never be encountered. We drill for, prevent, and are continually educated in managing fires. What do we know about other personal and disaster-related crises in the schools? What theoretical philosophies might apply? What research and what information that others have learned "the hard way" from experiencing crises might help schools prepare for crisis? How can we support young people in crisis who have previously been ignored?

These are the questions that this volume intends to address. It provides an update on the past 40 years of crisis intervention, an overview of techniques applicable within the school environment, and recommendations for approaches and necessary components in establishing a comprehensive preventive school district crisis intervention program.

If the reader has worked in the schools, unlike other agencies, she has probably found herself in several crisis-related roles. Since crisis intervention is a generic term, the following chapters divide school related crisis skills into four arenas:

1. Working directly with the individuals in crisis (e.g., suicidal students, behaviorally out-of-control students, victims of physical or sexual abuse).
2. Consulting with professionals who work with individuals in crisis (e.g., teachers, especially those of "at-risk" students, counselors, and principals).
3. Intervening during and just after a disaster when large numbers of staff and students are in crisis.
4. Consulting with administrators to develop a district-wide comprehensive crisis management system.

Information pertinent to delivery of direct crisis intervention services is presented together with information on consultation in the middle portion of this book, and intervention and organizational crisis planning are addressed in the final portion.

WHAT IS A CRISIS?

Implications of the "Crisis" Word

In day-to-day life, the term crisis takes on a multitude of connotations. Crisis at times appears to be something of a popular trend in our culture. We have personality crises, midlife crises, and identity crises. Turning 40 may precipitate a crisis; an automotive breakdown may result in a crisis; if the Florida fruit crop freezes, the evening news terms the event a crisis; internationally, the Iranian hostage situation was a crisis; when thousands of people died of starvation in Ethiopia, the ravages of famine constituted a crisis; and threat of nuclear war and destruction of the environment definitely qualify as crises.

Across the professional literature, terms such as crisis and crisis intervention also refer to a multiplicity of occurrences and events. In some articles, crisis implies an act of suicide; in others, it refers to the victims of disaster. Crisis intervention may turn out to be operationally defined as grief counseling, as managing the scene of a violent crime, or as physically apprehending someone.

As a concept, crisis has had a good deal of popular appeal, but as a construct, crisis has not established a core of meaning or formal theoretical base (Auerbach & Kilmann, 1987). As a clinical technique, crisis intervention consists of short-term, applied interventions that do not fall under the umbrella of traditional psychotherapy. Definition and formalization of technique have only begun quite recently (Aguilera & Messick, 1974; Caplan, 1964; McGee, 1974; Schulberg & Sheldon, 1968; Taplin, 1971).

Attempts at Formally Defining "Crisis"

Most attempts at a formal definition of "crisis" focus on the emotional state and perceptions of the individual(s) involved instead of the causal situation. One review (Auerbach & Kilmann, 1977) concluded, "across models there seems to be general agreement that crisis is a response state characterized by high levels of subjective discomfort at which the individual is at least temporarily unable to emit the overt or covert behaviors required to modify the stressfulness of his environment" (p. 1189). For example, Klein and Lindemann focused on the social mileu when they called crisis "the acute and often prolonged disturbance that may occur in an individual or social orbit as a result of an emotional hazard. The crisis of the individual is often a manifestation of a group crisis; conversely, the development of an interpersonal crisis may lead to a crisis situation for the group of which the individual is a significant member" (Klein and Lindemann, 1961, p. 284). Gerald Caplan called crisis "psychological disequilibrium in a person who confronts a hazardous circumstance that for him constitutes an important problem which he can, for the time being, neither escape nor solve with his customary problem solving resources" (Caplan, 1964, p. 53).

Other definitions include "any rapid change or encounter that is foreign to a person's usual experience" (Hansel, 1976).

Further attempts to define crisis have been made through symptomology: feelings of tiredness and exhaustion, helplessness, inadequacy, confusion, anxiety, and disorganization of functioning in work relationships (Halpern, 1973). Some researchers have posited symptoms of vulnerability, suggestability (Taplin, 1971), or reduced defensiveness (Halpern, 1973) with the precipitation of crisis. Finally, some theorists emphasize a breakdown in coping (Caplan, 1964; Lazarus, 1980) in which the individual in crisis feels he or she "is at the end of his rope, having tried everything he knows and can think of. He has finally succumbed" (Puryear, 1979, p. 49). Caplan (1964) wrote that the individual in crisis had exceeded his "homeostatic or equilibrium" capacities. This implies that a crisis is precipitated when a situation occurs that overloads coping skills and defense mechanisms. Therefore, an individual experiencing a crisis often sees the problem as hopeless because he or she cannot resolve the crisis with his or her customary problem-solving skills.

Lydia Rapoport (1962) added to the overall crisis concept by noting that a crisis can be precipitated by a loss, the threat of a loss, or a challenge. According to her conceptualization, perception plays a vital role in determining what is a crisis—that is, the importance or meaning to the individual. Loss of employment may be construed by one person as a crisis and by another as a cause for celebration.

What about an individual who "goes off the deep end" over an apparent minor incident? Sifneos (1960) has answered this question by outlining four factors that contribute to the crisis situation:

1. A hazardous event that leads to
2. A vulnerable state that is further aggravated by
3. A precipitating event that results in
4. An active state of crisis.

A student might have suffered through a nasty parental divorce 6 months ago. One day his dog runs away, and he begins to throw chairs in the classroom. Thus, the "straw that broke the camel's back" cannot be understood unless viewed in the context of previous life experiences.

A few points are consistent. One is that it is the perception of the individual that defines a crisis—not the event itself. Although some events, such as parental divorce or being victimized by violent crime, do commonly create crisis states for individuals, this is not necessarily the case. Other less commonly traumatic incidents are less universally crisis laden but hold the potential to be tremendous crisis inducers for some. Examples of such crisis inducers are the transition from home to school or being placed in a special education class.

A second point emphasized across these definitions is that the individual in crisis has a very difficult time negotiating life while in this crisis state, however brief that state is. He or she often is "taken over" by emotion and panic. Rational thought processes and objectivity in confronting and "thinking through" a problem are temporarily lost. In essence, he may need someone to provide the element of rationality for him while he gets back on his emotional feet. This emotionality and loss of rationality can be a much more complicated problem for children and adolescents, who often may not realize themselves that they are in a state of crisis (Sandoval, 1985).

A third point is that the crisis state is not seen, in itself, as psychopathology, nor is it chronic. However, crises can and usually do occur more frequently in those with chronic psychopathology or environmental stress problems. Thus, crisis is a "normal" reaction to an "abnormal" stressor that is generally resolved in a period of 6 weeks to 7 months (Lewis, Gottesman, & Gutstein, 1979). It is normal for a teacher to be shocked and upset subsequent to a violent attack; it is normal for children to be tearful and clinging following the death of a loved one.

However, it has been noted that cases of severe bereavement may take substantially longer (Lazarus, 1980).

This Book's Definition

For the purposes of this book, a crisis is defined as *an important and seemingly unsolvable problem with which those involved feel unable to cope* (Caplan, 1964; Smead, 1985). This definition would not rule out any of the scenarios of the preceding paragraphs. In actuality, it is difficult to limit the sorts of crises that may arise in the schools, for they cover the continuum between a first-year teacher's tears when her class is out of control to violent attacks in school halls. This definition also implies that what is a crisis to one individual may not be a crisis to another. What is a crisis today may be much more routinely managed in schools of the future.

WHAT HAPPENS IF CRISES ARE UNATTENDED?

A Brief Look at the Research

Many of the theorists in crisis intervention literature assume that long-term pathology can result from poorly resolved crises (Caplan, 1964; Golan, 1978; Puryear, 1979; Erickson, 1968). If the individual copes in a manner that is counterproductive in the long run (alcoholism, withdrawal, aggression, and, in the extreme, suicide), then he or she not only becomes entrenched in coping habits that are likely to perpetuate future crises but may also have difficulty negotiating the developmental tasks (Erickson, 1963) of that portion of his or her life. Another possibility is that the individual may "get stuck" in the crisis state, an alternative that could lead to serious long-term depression or psychological malfunctioning.

These assertions are based largely on clinical and informal case study data. In fact, there is not a great deal of conclusive research that establishes the effectiveness of crisis intervention practices (Auerbach & Kilmann, 1977). Since crisis is not a homogeneous or well-delineated concept, and since crisis intervention techniques vary on a number of factors (the service provider, the service recipient, the setting, the techniques), it is difficult to get an empirical "fix" on the big picture. A great deal of further research is required with regard to setting, technique, and specific goals.

The assertion that individuals who are sufficiently terrorized may lead a diminished or less effective life from that point on certainly presents with a good deal of face validity to those working in the schools. Experienced counselors, school psychologists, and teachers readily point to students who have never really functioned well since their parents were divorced, or to others who never really "got over" failing the fifth grade.

In fact, there is a relatively substantial body of research that documents a strong relationship between behavioral problems in school and crisis events in children's lives (see Cowen & Hightower, 1986, for a review). Events such as divorce, death of a significant other, and severe medical problems establish a much higher risk for school behavior problems, a risk that rises sharply with increased incidences of such crises. Researchers (Rutter, 1983) call for more specific information charting the adverse consequences associated with particular stressful events.

In general, authors and researchers in this area recommend not only immediate postcrisis treatment but treatment in advance to prevent as many adverse reactions as possible. Presently there are more specific interventions under scrutiny, such as those documenting the effectiveness of various treatment approaches in schools, especially those approaches directed at postdivorce intervention (Pedro-Carroll & Cowen, 1985; Stolberg & Garrison, 1985).

Age of the Child

Maccoby (1983) asserts that the younger a child is the more environmental support and structure he or she requires to weather a crisis without lasting emotional scars. Maccoby also notes that the younger the child, the greater the likelihood of behavioral problems or disorganization during a crisis. Logically, then, parents and professionals take on different roles for intervention as the child gets older: They assume active protectiontist sorts of roles for younger children and more supportive, ancillary roles for teens.

Crisis-Resistant Children?

A related and fascinating line of research emerging during the past decade is the study of the invulnerable, crisis-resistant child. Researchers observe children who have experienced quite profound levels of stress and crisis and have emerged apparently competent and well adjusted in spite of the experience (Garmezy, 1975, 1976, 1981, 1983; Garmezy, Masten, Nordstrom, & Ferrarese, 1979). Werner and Smith (1982) report in their 20-year longitudinal study of such children that about 1 in 10 appears to emerge from profound problems of physiology, poverty, and family instability unscathed. The three overall factors found to favor invincibility include:

1. Active, socially engaging, and autonomous personality from infancy.
2. Having someone within the family to offer genuine support and emotional closeness.
3. Significant peer and extrafamilial support (e.g., teachers, clergy, neighbors).

One cannot help supposing that such findings may someday give us clues regarding the design of preventive services that would reduce the emotional toll that many childhood crises have traditionally been associated with.

CRISIS SITUATIONS COMMONLY PRESENTING IN SCHOOLS

The numbers and severity of crises in schools generally appear to be increasing (National School Safety Center, 1988, 1989). Whatever the trend, any teacher will report that crisis-related problems are commonplace in preventing students from progressing educationally. Although few of us feel completely prepared to face and manage abuse, physical violence, or assaults, the simple reality is that most of us will, even those of us in "successful" schools and prominent neighborhoods (Jay, 1989).

Even in a rural midwest neighborhood school, crisis-related situations significant enough to interfere with children's educational progress have been shown to be quite commonplace (Wise & Smead, 1989). In one study, 123 teachers from three rural school districts in West Central Illinois were asked to report problems that interfered with their students' educational progress. In these small midwest communities, 63% of the teachers reported family members with alcohol or drug problems, 88% parents divorcing or separating, 48% student with drug or alcohol problems, 34% student getting seriously injured or ill, 17% student raped or otherwise physically attacked (nonfamily related), 28% suicide or suicide attempt of family member, 71% of the teachers reported child abuse or sexual abuse in the home.

Among those situations that teachers felt least able to intervene with were child/sexual abuse, major problems with parents, students involved with drugs or alcohol, divorce, and family substance abuse. These problems are obviously well outside the time and energy allotment, if not training, of the average teacher to attempt to manage. Yet it would be difficult for them to close their eyes to such difficulties in individuals with whom they are confronted day after day. Surely, working with students in crisis without help from support staff leads not only to loss of student progress but also to teacher burnout and ultimate loss of teaching staff (Hazelwood, 1989).

What follows is a review of various crises occurring or manifesting themselves frequently in the school arena. Any school personnel who have been working for a few years have probably seen every one of them. Available statistics provide the reader with some frame of reference regarding what we know of relative frequencies of various possible crisis situations in the schools.

Violent Crimes

In general, violent crime in the schools appears to be fairly frequent, although there is some conflict regarding the severity of the problem or whether it is increasing (McDermott, 1984). Clearly, however, the topic is a matter of concern to the general public, The Gallup Poll on the Public's attitudes toward the public schools identifies discipline as the number-one concern in all but 1 year since 1969.

During the late 1970s and the 1980s there has been a general uproar concerning crime and violence in schools (National School Safety Center, 1988, 1989). In 1978 the National Institute of Education published *Violent Schools—Safe Schools: The Safe School Study Report to the Congress.* The findings suggested relatively high rates of crime in schools across the country. During each month:

- Approximately 25% of schools are vandalized.
- One in 100 schools experiences a bomb threat in a typical month.
- More than 2.4 million secondary school students are victims of theft, many involving force, weapons, and threats.
- Nearly 282,000 students are attacked in schools, with younger students being the most likely victims.
- About 130,000 of the 1.1 million secondary school teachers have something of value stolen.
- Approximately 5,200 teachers report being physically attacked; they are five times as likely as students to be seriously injured in those attacks (National School Boards Association, 1981, 1984).

What is more, these figures are probably conservative underestimates. The N.I.E. study probably understated the actual incidence of school violence because approximately two-thirds of personal thefts and robberies and almost three-fourths of property damages go unreported to the police (Toby, 1984). Secretary of Education T. H. Bell has since reported that crime in the schools has increased steadily since these 1978 statistics.

Government figures for 1985 documented 450,000 violent crimes in our nation's schools and colleges. Assaults accounted for most of the incidents, followed by robbery and rape (Mayfield, 1986). Keen (1989) noted that 3 million children are attacked at school each year and that weapons are used in 70,000 assaults. A startling (50%) increase has been cited in the number of attacks on teachers from 1973 to 1985 (McEvoy, 1988a).

The national statistics appear to hold up quite well in local reports of school crime. For example, a study of Boston's public schools (Fox, 1983) indicated:

- Thirty-three percent of the students admitted carrying weapons to school.
- Half of the teachers and almost 40% of the students were victims of school robbery, assault, or larceny.
- Nearly 40% of students reported that they feared for their safety in school or reported avoiding corridors and rest rooms.

It is interesting to note that FBI statistics indicate that children under the age of 15 were responsible for 381 murders in 1985 as well as 2,645 rapes, 18,021 aggravated assaults, and 13,899 robberies. What's more, only 7% of the population was responsible for all these crimes. Youth homicide has doubled in the last 20 years (McEvoy, 1988a). These are serious, habitual juvenile offenders. And more frequently than in the past, they attend school.

Although it is difficult to know precisely how overall youth crime statistics affect the school, one can assume that the overall sense of physical and emotional safety in schools has been compromised. Even if youth crime is conservatively construed as beyond school-based in-tervention, experts across the nation point to schools as the primary setting in which to control it. Thus, as with many crisis-laden situations, the schools may not be part of the problem, but they become an impor-tant element in the solution. Early prevention appears to be the most effective way to stem juvenile delinquency and drug activity. Of direct import to educators is the growing sense that to control this wave of juvenile activity collaborative efforts among educators, law enforcers, and community members will probably be indispensable (National School Safety Center, 1989). Early prevention programs, strategies, and curricula aimed at grades 3, 4, and 5 appear to show the most promise.

Certainly many other forms of violent crime occur that potentially affect educational progress. For example, Memmot and Stone (1989) report that one child is killed every day in accidental shootings, and ten more are injured.

Everything from family violence to automobile accidents that upset a child's life can intrude into the school setting. Although it is not practical to list them exhaustively in the context of this book, one can speculate: the variety is endless.

Teacher Victimization

Approximately 5,200 teachers are the victims of violence at school each month, and attacks on teachers doubled between 1973 and 1985 (Mc-Evoy, 1988a). What could prevent teachers from being victimized? What do teachers need to recover from these incidents? How can the schools support them? These are among the questions now being asked by educators and administrators nationwide.

Child and Adolescent Depression and Suicide

In addition to violent crime and accidental shootings, child and adolescent suicide has also evidenced dramatic increases. The incidence of teen-age suicide appears to have tripled since 1955 and doubled since 1970 (Vidal, 1986); it is presently cited as the second leading cause of death for teen-agers, with accidents as the primary cause. It is difficult to get accurate figures on the incidence of teen suicide, but recent governmental figures indicate that approximately 5,000 young people in the 15- to 24-year-old age group commit suicide each year. As many as a third of teen-agers reported having seriously thought of suicide, and 14% report actually having attempted it (Friend, 1988). Historically the schools have been reluctant to play an active role involving intervention vis-à-vis the suicide problem. Recently, however, Dr. Scott Poland (1990a) has outlined more active roles for schools, including:

- To detect potentially suicidal students.
- To assess the severity level of the suicidal student.
- To notify the parents of a suicidal student.
- To work with the parents to secure the needed supervision and services for the student.
- To monitor the student and provide ongoing assistance.

Child and Adolescent Depression

Dr. Donald H. McKnew, Jr., a child psychiatrist affiliated with the National Institute of Mental Health, estimates that from 3 to 6 million children are in need of clinical help for depression. These children are represented across all economic levels. An estimated 10% of all children between the ages of 6 and 12 have experienced depression severe enough to interfere with their everyday functioning, such as going to school. Further, about half of these youngsters dwell on committing suicide. The symptoms they exhibit are much the same as have been documented with adults:

- Difficulty sleeping and eating appropriately.
- Pervasive feeling of hopelessness and helplessness.
- Difficulty concentrating, lethargy, and difficulty completing tasks.
- Withdrawal.
- Anger, aggressiveness, and poor social adjustment.
- Low self-esteem: self-deprecating remarks, extreme sensitivity to making mistakes, repeatedly behaving in a manner that brings about negative consequences for themselves.

Recent research suggests that some childhood depression may be endogenous or "inborn" physiologically based depression and that the pattern may begin as early as a few years of age. The cyclic pattern of depression will result in snowballing of symptoms if it is not treated.

Divorce, Death, or Other Major Losses

Almost anyone who works in schools in any role has experienced children in crisis following their parents' divorce. It is not surprising, therefore, to note that there are so many children suffering through a divorce in any one typical elementary school at any one time that counselors frequently can have ongoing divorce groups that run throughout the school year. By now most mental health professionals are familiar with the basic statistics: one in two marriages ends in divorce, and at least 1 million children are involved in divorce proceedings *every year*. This represents a 100% increase since 1954. Moreover, the "average" or "typical" family today is no longer the nuclear family, since the majority of American children live in single-parent families or blended (step) families (King & Goldman, 1988).

Although some of these families seek outside help and support for children, at least as many do not. Since divorce seems to create a temporary interruption in their parents' ability to parent, the most stable aspect of a child's life lies in the classroom. It is not unusual for the classroom to be the "safest" place to act out emotional upset and family turbulence: withdrawal, tearfulness, or aggression. Any of these patterns interrupts the child's ability to benefit from education, and it interferes with the progress of the rest of the class, creating stress for everyone.

Death or loss of someone close can also precipitate crisis. This happens most frequently when the new loss is coupled with previous losses and when day-to-day family functioning breaks down subsequent to the death or other major losses.

Mistreated Children

Mistreatment includes physical/sexual abuse, neglect, and psychological abuse. The House Select Committee on Children, Youth, and Families found that the number of abused or neglected children increased by 54.9% between 1981 and 1985, with child sexual abuse rising the fastest (57.4%) of all. It is estimated that abuse of one form or another is administered to nearly 2 million children each year. For anyone who has worked in the schools, these statistics document what we already know: mistreatment, even severe mistreatment, is not unusual, and in any school there are a number of children for whom physical, sexual, or emotional abuse is seriously suspected to be interfering with the child's development and learning. Some of the most compelling long-term crisis situations that I have seen have been cases of children living with ongoing mistreatment. One student, Andrea, presently 20 years old, called me to explain why she had spent so much time in the counselor's and psychologist's office in high school. Throughout high school Andrea was experiencing one crisis after another: suicide note after suicide note, tearful day after tearful day. It was not until she was out of her parents' home, however, that she dared to confess the underlying, ongoing problem that had plagued her all those years. Apparently her father had been forcing sex with her since she was 12. As is not unusual, her mother did not interfere and, in fact, acted to prevent any knowledge of this from escaping the family. Presently Andrea attends individual and group therapy sessions, lives independently, and is working on putting together positive, healthy relationships. This story is not unusual; in our experience students referred for psychological services in the schools are very commonly, often 50% of the time, victims of abuse, usually sexual abuse. This clinical "hunch" is supported by national statistics.

In the 1981 National Study (USDHHS, 1981), the incidence of sexual exploitation was reported at 0.7 per 1,000 individuals. Compiled results from a number of studies (Germain, Brassard, & Hart, 1985) suggest that 20–35% of women and 10–18% of men have reported sexual encounters with an adult. Typically the abuser was from within the family (75%) or someone the child knew (90%) (Finkelhor, 1981).

Approximately 60,000 cases of physical abuse are reported each year in the United States (Gelles & Straus, 1979). The 1981 National Study reported an incidence of 3.4 per 1,000 for physical abuse and 1.7 per 1,000 for physical neglect (USDHHS, 1981).

Obviously psychological mistreatment or abuse is more difficult to document and count. However, this same study reported an incidence of 2.2 per 1,000 children and emotional neglect at 1.0 per 1,000 children.

The incidence of reported episodes of child abuse has grown steadily over the past few decades. Probably this trend represents recent efforts at raising consciousness and protecting children's rights rather than actual increases in abuse. However, the mere fact that children are more aware and assertive regarding the reporting of child abuse increases the responsibility and involvement of the school district: the majority of calls are made by school staff. Not only does this increasing trend require additional time to complete and file reports and to allow for consultation with child protection personnel, but teachers and counselors are also faced with coping with additional "fallout" from the families and with the very big quandry of where their responsibility with a particular child ends. Does the teacher mention the incident again? What if there appears to be further abuse but there is not evidence to make a case?

Many times cases of sexual or psychological abuse are difficult to prove or document. Can we ignore those cases for which substantial evidence is not available to force therapy or maintain a case with the child welfare department? Many of these children and adolescents are in ongoing crisis, often tearful in school, and they threaten self-destruction. Sadly, we cannot stop or interfere with the abusive or neglectful family in many cases; perhaps support through the crisis might be our moral duty in addition to education to prevent the well-known tendency for child-abuse victims to become criminals or abusers themselves.

Identification of a Handicapped Child

Any psychologist working in education is likely to encounter the very difficult situation of confronting relatively unsuspecting parents with the unwelcome news that their child is functioning with a handicap, sometimes a severe one. The severe emotional reaction commonly associated with this shock is often sufficient to send a family into a crisis state. We should have been trained well to cope with this particular crisis, but all too often support is lacking among school personnel, and adversarial relationships are spawned during this initial shock of recognition. Most times even basic support, such as a staffing prior to the formal meeting announcing assessment results, allowing parents to observe alternative placement settings, allowing parents to participate appropriately in the assessment itself, connecting parents with community resources such as parent support groups, and "second opinions" if necessary, may go a long way toward preventing a crisis during this process. If we can learn to recognize this time as a likely candidate for crisis induction and employ crisis intervention techniques when appropriate, perhaps we could then establish the best relationship with parents from the very beginning of their interaction with the special education system.

Disasters

Traditionally schools have prepared for a handful of disasters known to beset the community: fires, floods, blizzards, and so forth. Modern conditions are adding many more to the list: AIDS, bomb threats, chemical spills, sniper attacks, violent intruders, and terrorism, to name a few. No community seems to be immune to these kinds of calamities, and the National Associations of School Principals are increasingly calling for school plans to manage the immediate event and also to support students dealing with the long-term psychological shocks they receive.

WHY ARE SCHOOL CRISES MORE COMMON TODAY?

What ever happened to good, old-fashioned discipline? Aren't kids the same as they used to be? Are we just getting too soft? Whereas the threat of detention, or a talk with a given authority figure can solve behavior or motivational problems for emotionally well-adjusted kids from stable families and communities, these methods simply don't solve problems many children in our society are presently facing. What is it about our society that has changed so dramatically? Many professionals believe that stress has increased tremendously in society because of increases in change itself. Society moves much faster than it used to. Families move, break up, and regroup with other families. Communities change, schools relocate, a favorite restaurant could close next week, a favorite route home from work may be wiped out by a new freeway. It has been quite well established that change—even positive change—creates stress. Increased stress increases the risk of crisis. The following issues have contributed in a major way to much of the crisis climate we now so frequently encounter in schools.

Changes in the Mental Health System

Alternatives to inpatient psychiatric hospitalization have decreased the numbers of individuals who remain in residential facilities both briefly and chronically (Polak & Kirby, 1976). As our mental health technology improves, our focus more and more is on community treatment of all psychological disabilities. When individuals between 2 and 21 years of age move to the community, they also move to community schools. Depending on the location of state facilities or private facilities vis-à-vis your school district, you may have already noticed indications of this trend. Children previously placed residentially in a state hospital or school are moving to less restrictive half-way houses or back home with families (with, it is hoped, additional support for the parents).

Private facilities are also less of an option than they have been in the past. Skyrocketing medical expenses have led most insurance companies to restrict the number of days per year an individual may spend in an inpatient setting. Thus, very few families have the financial option of maintaining a child in a residential setting.

The end result of all of these trends is that more children and adolescents with the most severe disabilities are coming to school, thereby increasing the potential for a host of crises: violent physical and emotional outbursts (common in autistic, mentally retarded, and emotionally/behaviorally disturbed students), suicidal behavior (emotionally/behaviorally disturbed students), and many other actions that are generally a challenge to the educational system (e.g., truancy, drug abuse).

To complicate matters further, a significant amount of evidence indicates that children and adolescent populations in this country have been severely underserved in the area of community mental health services for decades (Danzy, 1989; see next section). The public sector has reduced these services even further since the 1960s. All in all, the chances are that movement to community services will not necessarily be accompanied by the necessary community support services, especially in the area of crisis intervention. Once again, the school may be the only mental health service the child and family have.

Unmet Mental Health Needs

The need for increased mental health services to children and adolescents has been recognized for more than 20 years (Danzy, 1989). In 1969 the Joint Commission on Mental Health of Children reported to the Congress that mental illness among children had risen 150% during the previous 10 years. It was estimated that in the United States there were 4 million emotionally disturbed children. In addition, 15 states had no public or private facilities for mental health treatment of children, and 24 states had no public facilities for children from low- and middle-income populations in need of mental health care.

In 1978 the President's Commission on Mental Health found that more than half of the nation's population was comprised of children, adolescents, and the elderly in need of mental health care, but these populations were receiving the fewest mental health services. The priority recommendation was to increase the number of professionals trained to work with these special populations.

There is substantial evidence, however, that we are not meeting these needs even today. The District of Columbia Mental Health Association reported in 1975 that approximately 20,000 residents under age 18 were in need of mental health services, and 5,700 of that population were suffering from severe emotional disturbances. Again in 1984, a survey report (Banik, 1984) estimated that approximately 22,000 children under the age of 18 were in need of mental health services.

Even though large numbers of children appear to be in need of mental health services, there are consistently low numbers of qualified professionals available to work with them on either an outpatient or inpatient basis. School psychology is no exception. In 1989 there were unfilled positions for school psychologists across the country. The state of Texas recently conducted a study of school children with emotional problems and found that a huge portion of that population was not identified or receiving appropriate services (Texas Education Agency, 1987). This underidentification occurred especially in districts that had no psychologists in their employ.

Changes in Educational Policy

Ever since the now familiar federal mandate PL 94-142, was passed some 15 years ago, we have been educating children with all disabilities in the public schools and doing so in less and less restrictive educational settings. This policy, of course, increased the numbers of crisis-prone students in the schools.

The increase in expense of residential settings has further pressured schools to provide an appropriate education to handicapped students within their own school districts. It is far less expensive to hire a teacher a one-on-one basis for a student than to send him or her off to a more isolated setting.

The national trend continues to move in the direction of including more "at-risk" student populations in schools. The juvenile justice establishment is focusing nationally on alternatives to expulsion, which rest primarily in alternative programs in or under guidance from the public schools.

Substance Abuse

According to the 19th Annual Gallup Poll of the Public's Attitudes Toward Public Schools, for the second year in a row, the public in 1987 ranked drug abuse first and lack of discipline second as the biggest problems facing schools today.

Children are found to be taking a drink of alcohol at a younger age than ever before, with some starting as early as 5 years. A recent survey of 500,000 children between the ages of 9 and 12 suggested that about half had experienced peer pressure to try drugs or alcohol. The National Institute of Drug Abuse notes that in today's society it is not uncommon to find children at age 9 or 10 regularly using marijuana or alcohol.

In a recent national survey of drug abuse among high school seniors, more than half (57%) of American teen-agers said they have used illicit drugs at least once before completing high school. This survey further noted that many of these teen-agers (40%) had used an illicit drug in the past year, and one-fourth of them had used another substance besides marijuana.

Marijuana continues to be the most widely used drug: half of the seniors reported using it at some time during their lifetime, and 3.3% reported using it daily. However, use of marijuana does appear to be dropping off; since the beginning of the survey in 1978, the lowest percentage of seniors ever (36%) reported using it in the last year (University of Michigan, 1987).

A recent drop (from 12.7% to 10.3% was also reported in the use of cocaine in 1987, which was the first drop since the beginning of the survey. A decrease of about one-third (from 6.2% in 1986 to 4.3% in 1987) was apparent in the number of seniors who claimed to be "current users" of cocaine (National Institute of Drug Abuse, 1985).

This overall trend does not appear to be present, however, in the case of crack cocaine. It is cheap and highly addictive. Even when casually watching the evening news or glancing over any newspaper, one cannot but notice that any reporting of recent crime among adolescents or adults is continually linked to the soaring use of crack. Many urban adolescents have become involved in drug trafficking. Some attend school equipped with electronic pagers and are earning vast amounts of money dealing crack on school campuses. In an effort to shut this sort of activity down, a new federal "schoolyard law" was passed recently that imposes stiffer penalties for adults convicted of selling or distributing drugs within 1,000 feet of a school.

Teen-age alcohol abuse is another national concern. The trend of teen-age alcohol abuse shows no signs of decreasing in recent years. Whereas nearly all Michigan seniors reported experience with drinking (92%), more than a third (38%) reported having five or more drinks in a row on at least one occasion within the previous 2 weeks. Although estimates of teenagers involved with alcohol remain at a fairly constant rate of 90%, some research (Georgia Task Force on Alcohol, 1987) indicates that 19% of sixth graders reported using alcohol.

Further, we know that substance abuse is linked with other sorts of crisis behavior such as suicide (West, 1984): approximately 40% to 90% of adolescents who attempted suicide had been drinking at the time. Violent and criminal behaviors are also linked with substance abuse, and at times it has been argued that behavioral patterns predispose individuals to substance abuse rather than substance abuse assuming primary responsibility for the inappropriate behavioral patterns or loss of coping as ordinarily supposed.

Instability in the Traditional Nuclear Family

Estimates presently suggest that 30–50% of children in American homes live with a single parent. Currently in the United States only one in five families includes a father as the breadwinner and a mother working in the home with children. Whereas this situation is not in itself unstable or unhealthy, single-parent familes are at risk for a multitide of crisis-related problems. Often this parent is operating without the traditional support systems of extended family members, and very often this family is living on an income that is below poverty level—a startling 60% of single-parent families now live on poverty incomes. Freese (1984) indicated the broken-home problem of divorce and separated parents: 75% of suicidal teen-agers come from one-parent homes; another 15% had a parent who was away for long periods. About 30% of the youth were not living with either parent at the time they attempted suicide.

Families also are more mobile than ever before. Not only does this frequently cut them off from extended family support, but all the changes associated with frequent moves can be overwhelming to some children. Glasser (1969) emphasized moving from one community to a new one as a cause of anger and frustration among children and adolescents.

A number of researchers have found abuse related to stress of parenting, with stress-producing factors including the birth of several children close together and special physical or emotional problems. With the increasing isolation of the nuclear family from relatives and with the increasing number of one-parent families, parents do not get a break or support.

Violent families have always existed, but now people talk more about them. Children speak up, and wives are less concerned about confiding in school personnel. Characteristics that do not change are that (1) community resources are not sufficient to meet the needs of battered families, (2) usually the children and wife remain with a violent or abusive situation in the long run, and (3) most times, the individual perpetuating the violence denies the problem and refuses to seek help (Barnes, 1989). Since police rarely file reports on domestic violence and even more rarely arrest men for battering, the chances of apprehension generally are slim. For example, Cleveland police received about 15,000 domestic violence calls during a 9-month period. Reports were filed on 700 of these cases, and arrests were made on 460, or on about one of every 32 calls (Ohio Attorney General, 1979). Chances are these children are going to live with violence until they are old enough to fight back, run, or move away. They need support from somewhere, and they are not likely to get it from community mental health agencies, even when we encourage them to do so.

Day Care

The House Committee on Children, Youth, and Families estimates that 7 million children presently are being raised in day-care facilities. The committee also found that the great majority of these facilities are not licensed and do not provide any structured activities for children. The kids are generally left to entertain themselves.

In addition to children in day care, another 7 million children are left alone after school while their parents are at work. The experts continue to assess possible adverse consequences of "latchkey" children left on their own; few of them would suggest that this situation is productive. Many older children are left with the further responsibility for their younger siblings. Thus, children increasingly are left to be "independent adults" at day care and home. They are faced with the confusing notion, however, that when they arrive at school they are to follow directions and structure.

Television Violence

Although television has traditionally been accused of cultivating "undesirable" attitudes and behavior, questions regarding the impact of hours and hours of violence witnessed on television are being taken more and more seriously across the nation. Confusion and anger over the noncommittal Surgeon General's report *Television and Growing Up: The Impact of Televised Violence* has led to a generalized recognition among social scientists and government officials that television has been shown to be one of the several significant contributors to aggressive and antisocial attitudes and behavior (Liebert, Sprafkin, & Davidson, 1982).

Over decades (1956–1976) of television viewing and 67 major studies on the relationship between TV violence and aggressive behavior, the arguments rage on. Of all the studies, the final tally was that 77% of the work revealed an association, 20% no results, and about 3% an inverse association. More rigorous experimental studies were more likely to yield results indicating a positive association (Andison, 1977).

Even if television influences children in the mildest of ways, the sheer volume of exposure makes the possibilities quite frightening. This is so first because the sheer number of hours the typical child spends before the television set is impressive: between 2 and 4 hours per day for individuals between the ages of 4 and 20 years (Comstock, Chaffee, Katzman, McCombs, & Roberts, 1978). Second, it appears nearly impossible to avoid viewing violence, especially for children and adolescents. The percentage of all programs exhibiting violence between 1967 and 1979 ranged from 73% (mean of five violent acts per program) to 89% (mean of six violent acts per program). Over daytime weekend hours (prime time for younger children, of course) for the same period, nearly all programs contained violence (91–100%), with a mean number of violent acts per program around six (Signorielli, Gross, & Morgan, 1982).

HISTORY AND FUNDAMENTAL CONCEPTS OF CRISIS INTERVENTION

Rigorous research regarding crisis is a tremendous challenge since, by definition, one cannot predict or control where a crisis will occur. Thus, the traditional scientific approach including a priori hypotheses, isolation of one or two significant variables, and experimental controls is rarely, if ever, an option. Ad hoc explanations and recollections together with clinical experience presently make up the lion's share of our present body of literature and are generally the best we can do in the way of data collection. Thus, general incidence data, case studies, and borrowing from what we, as psychologists, know about human behavior in general make up the bulk of sources of useful information.

Some empirical data have been gleaned from studies of human reaction to an extremely stressful event including coping with the trauma of surgery, concentration camps, sudden death of spouses and relatives, slow death of a child, and disasters (Baker & Chapman, 1962; Holmes & Rahe, 1967). Further, a number of studies have attempted to measure the effectiveness of crisis intervention techniques but have been impeded by the "uniformity assumption" that recipients of crisis intervention are a homogeneous group and that crisis intervention represents a uniform treatment delivered in the same manner by individuals who are not different from each other (Auerbach & Kilmann, 1977). In reality, crisis intervention techniques are a cluster of services that vary according to location, characteristics of recipients, characteristics of service delivery, etc. It is very difficult to put together a global evaluation of crisis intervention in any quasiscientific manner.

Early History

Slaikeu (1984) provides a comprehensive overview of the development of crisis intervention techniques and theory. Some of the trends that he notes are direct lineage to the development of crisis intervention in the schools that appears yet to be in its very beginning stages. To trace the beginning of crisis intervention is also to trace the beginnings of such mental health fundamentals as prevention of mental illness, community psychology, brief therapy, and telephone hotlines.

The study of crisis consistently is identified with the largest single building fire in history some 40 years ago in Boston. Nearly 500 people were killed in the Coconut Grove nightclub before the blaze was extinguished. Eric Lindemann and the Massachusetts General Hospital staff subsequently worked with both the survivors and the families. He published his reactions to this crisis treatment in an article titled "Symptomatology and Management of Acute Grief," which appeared in the September 1944 issue of *The American Journal of Psychiatry*. His writings reviewed the ongoing symptoms of the survivors over time as they adapted psychologically to the trauma (Lindemann, 1944).

During the 1950s Gerald Caplan joined Lindemann at the Wellesley Human Relations Center. Caplan, however, differentiated between personal crisis, such as those studied by Lindemann, and developmental crises. Developmental crises were predictable developmental "tasks" occurring at critical junctures in life. Caplan adopted Erickson's (1963) concepts of lifetime development as times of anticipated developmental crisis. Caplan looked at personal crises related to the negotiation of these stages. He noted that during or just after a personal crisis individuals appeared less able to cope with or negotiate the developmental demands in their lives, which in turn could lead to long-term disorganization or even mental illness. Since developmental crises could be anticipated, they could be prevented. If they could be prevented, probably some mental illness could be prevented, especially if it were sparked by these crisis situations. Thus, the concept of preventive mental health was born.

The focus of preventive mental health services was to work with community professionals including school counselors, nurses, and teachers on how to detect and help individuals through life crises in the community. Mental health consultation, much of what we would like school psychologists to be involved with, was born together with the primary ideological base for community psychology.

Pioneers in community psychology and brief preventive treatment built on these early ideas. Beginnings of crisis intervention in the 1940s and 1950s were catapulted into everyday application in 1963 when Congress passed the Community Mental Health Centers Act. Mental health services were no longer restricted to hospitals. Individuals in need could receive a wide range of affordable mental health care in a nearby neighborhood center. One of the community services mandated to be provided by these centers was 24-hour emergency or crisis care. Minor problems were emphasized as the treatment focus designed to prevent escalation of mental illness resulting from inability to constructively manage a crisis. During the 1960s the professional literature exploded with articles and books about crisis intervention theory and practice.

Modern traditions such as 24-hour hotlines (Slaikeu, 1984) and the use of paraprofessional and nonprofessional volunteers (McGee, 1974) became widespread across the country. The modern flourish of the brief psychotherapy literature for family therapy (see, for example, Haley, 1976) and for grief counseling and grief therapy (Worden, 1982) had its early roots in the new preventive psychology.

A second emphasis was placed on evaluation of these services, and a great body of literature has grown from program evaluation of community mental health centers (Baldwin, 1979; Butcher & Koss, 1978; Butcher & Maudal, 1976; Smith, 1977). As noted earlier, however, it is difficult to reach any overall conclusions regarding the effectiveness of crisis intervention or even various crisis intervention techniques because of confounds in experimental designs (Auerbach & Kilmann, 1977).

With the application of newly developed psychotropic medications and "dangerous to self or others" terms of commitment being adopted by most states, residential facilities began to empty. As a consequence, portions of the chronic psychiatric population began living longer segments of their lives in the community.

The recession of the 1970s together with more conservative political patterns in the 1980s underscored and applauded concepts in community psychology. Short-term therapy techniques became the only cost-effective alternative for many mental health budgets that were increasingly losing their funding. Some research (Cummings, 1977) suggested that short-term therapy was more effective than long-term psychotherapy, especially in light of the preventive aspect of the treatment. Further, the necessity of limiting psychotherapeutic treatment to coordinate with the financial limits of insurance agencies and individuals appeared appealing.

During the development of preventive community treatment in the

1960s, it would have been difficult to foresee the mushrooming need for such services 20 years later. With the tremendous increase in the incidence of crisis in the past few decades, the now traditional mental health system is overwhelmed. Emphasis on community treatment of widespread mental health problems such as substance abuse, dropping out of school, and violence is now not merely an alternative treatment but the sole realistic treatment option our society has.

Crises that presented in the community mental health center and hospitals to social workers, physicians, and clinical psychologists were very much the same as those that arose in the schools. Many times, the observant teacher had the very first opportunity to identify a potential crisis in the early years of a child's/family's life, before the family, and certainly the community, began to experience it. The idea of psychologists working in the schools in a preventive, consultative mode was a novel concept, especially in contrast with the more traditional testing roles of the educational psychologist. Thus, paralleling the growth of community emphasis and focus on prevention, a major genesis of school psychology and mental health consultation evolved.

Theoretical Assumptions

The concept of short-term crisis therapy is quite new (Aguilera & Messick, 1974; Caplan, 1964; McGee, 1974; Schulberg & Sheldon, 1968), and as an applied technique, it does not fall under traditional psychotherapy. It is important to emphasize yet again that the therapeutic approach to counseling and managing those in crisis is based on theoretical assumptions that are in stark contrast with the more traditional and long-term therapeutic approaches. Bits of theory and technique generally have evolved from applied, first-hand experience working with individuals in crisis rather than through an integrated conceptual base or theory. The backgrounds of individuals involved in this evolution have been quite interdisciplinary within the mental health professional umbrella.

It is not surprising, then, that crisis intervention techniques are loosely organized and include a variety of practical procedures. Overall characteristics of the approach include "reality-based" (e.g., practical) suggestions for getting through the immediate problem (Caplan, 1964), repeated contacts over a short time, and high therapist activity to help access available supports to promote readjustment or a return to the "normal" functioning of the individual (Caplan & Grunebaum, 1967). Any techniques that can be applied to this end usually qualify as crisis intervention techniques.

Therefore, crisis intervention skills used on a crisis hotline or adult clinic will almost certainly vary in substantial ways from those appropriate to children in a school environment. To date, school psychology has only barely begun to assemble a "little black bag" of useful methods for managing crises in schools. The following two sections expand on this "bag" of methods. However, it is important first to review the overarching, unifying concepts of the very heterogeneous field of crisis intervention.

First, reactions to crises such as feelings of helplessness and anxiety are thought to be normal rather than pathological. It is a normal reaction to a very abnormal situation or a very severe stressor. Second, techniques are focused on returning the individual to his or her "normal" or "precrisis" state as quickly as possible. The intent here is not to restructure personality as in more traditional psychotherapy.

The third point is related to the first two: the therapy or intervention is basically short-term. The more or less paralyzing emotional reactions to the crisis is assumed to be a reasonably temporary state. (Caplan suggests approximately 6 weeks for most crises, although there is some suggestion that serious cases of bereavement may extend for years.) Helping methods are characterized by repeated brief contacts with the individual during this time.

Fourth, attempts are made to avoid encouragement of ongoing dependency on the service provider. The individual in crisis is encouraged to use the ongoing, appropriate supports available to him or her in the community to resolve the current crisis and to avoid future crises: these include counseling centers, friends and family, financial aid, etc. While the individual remains in crisis, the crisis interventionist takes a much more active role if necessary than in traditional psychotherapy to help the client access these community supports.

The area of crisis intervention by the original theoretical design and also in practice over the past 20 years is truely multidisciplinary, with paraprofessionals and volunteers frequently involved in all phases of crisis intervention. This is in keeping with the philosophy that crises can be kept small if caught immediately by those on the "front lines." Thus, the role of teachers, counselors, nurses, and hotline volunteers is absolutely essential in the crisis context.

The more flexible and socially supported the person's coping strategies are, the greater the chance the individual can avoid the crisis state. Children and adolescents can only be assumed to manage crisis situations as well as their parents and families.

Fifth, people in crisis are more receptive to outside help because they have exhausted their own resources. Thus, the kind of help such people receive during this crucial time can exert a strong influence on the crisis outcome.

Stages of Crisis Development

What predictably happens when human beings encounter a crisis phenomenon? And how can knowing the sequence of events help us better
prepare ourselves and our society for crises? Caplan introduced many of
the seminal answers to these questions in his 1964 book *Principles of
Preventive Psychiatry*. In this work, Caplan introduces several seminal
concepts that have stood the tests of time.

First, Caplan noted that when a crisis occurs the events preceding and
following occur in four predictable stages.

Phase 1

There is an initial rise in tension or anxiety caused by a traumatic (crisis)
event. The individual finds himself faced with a problem that is ex-
ceedingly troubling because none of the problem-solving techniques,
rationalizations, or coping mechanisms that allowed the individual to
cope previously "work" in the present situation. This may be because the
individual has never previously faced this sort of loss, conflict, or dis-
appointment before (e.g., Denise is told by Tom, her husband of 12
years, that he is filing for divorce), or it may result from sudden forced
recognition of a previously denied circumstance (e.g., the Joneses receive information suggesting that their young child is handicapped). In
this phase, however, the individuals are not yet in crisis. The rise in
anxiety generally promotes a number of activities designed to avoid the
feared result: Denise convinces her husband to go into therapy to work
out differences. The Joneses take their child to a nationally recognized
clinic for a second opinion.

Phase 2

In the face of the continued impact of the stressing event, the attempts
made at problem solving are without success. Denise's husband begins to
skip therapy sessions and spends less and less time in the home. Overt
conflict breaks out frequently as Denise has difficulty containing her
anger at his behavior. The school informs Denise that her first-grade son
is experiencing behavior problems and refuses to complete his work.
The Joneses are told that the original diagnosis of mental retardation is
confirmed despite the child's apparent normal motor development.

Phase 3

During the third phase anxiety rises even higher. The individual ex-
hausts all possible resources, even those involving quite extreme means.

Denise begins to spend more time with her parents, including weekends in their home. She seeks help from the school counselor for her son and consults several attorneys regarding her legal rights under divorce. She begins to locate housing that she can afford on her own. The Joneses seek out third and fourth opinions, including neuropsychological batteries and MRI scans to determine precisely what is medically causing the symptoms their child is exhibiting or whether it is merely an erroneous product of school tests.

At this point, if the individuals involved are able to shift the goals of their coping, as Denise did, a crisis may be averted. Individuals operating alone, without support personnel, may not be able to manage this. In this latter case, the individual progresses to the fourth phase, which is active crisis.

Phase 4

Tension mounts to the breaking point, and severe emotional disorganization results (Caplan, 1964). The individual has exhausted his or her own internal strength, and social support is lacking. Following our examples, Denise was able to avert the crisis by using her own social support systems and by shifting her goals to begin to focus on establishing an independent life for herself.

The Joneses, however, push steadfastly forward but without success in their efforts to avoid crisis. Frequent calls to John's parents, who live out of state, result in confirmation that nothing could be "wrong" with John, Jr. They are told that when John senior was younger, there was also a period when he was somewhat slow to begin speaking, and he turned out to be fine. Medical bills began to tax their financial status. Marital difficulties begin to escalate under the pressure. Mr. Jones insists that their son should continue in regular kindergarten. Mrs. Jones feels extra help might not hurt and that possibly the child might be a little behind other children. When the medical tests turn up negative. Mrs. Jones takes John, Jr. to an out-of-state early childhood program that promises to remediate slow speech development and bizarre behavior. She does so without consulting her husband, since he has been sullen and withdrawn recently, further threatening their already fragile economic and emotional status. When she returns 4 weeks later, her child has progressed by only a few words, and his behavior has become much more difficult for her to control. Mr. Jones becomes frustrated and leaves. Mrs. Jones cries frequently, is not working, has few friends or family, and has exhausted her own ideas of what could be done next. She stays home not knowing what the next day will bring or how long she can manage to maintain present living accommodations. She seems unable to make a move to cope with the situation or to problem solve. It is when she receives her eviction notice that she tearfully explains her situation to the counselor at her son's elementaty school.

Outcome of Crisis

Crisis theory as elaborated by Caplan (1964), Erikson (1962, 1968), and Hill (1958) includes three possible outcomes of crisis: better than, similar to, or worse than precrisis functioning. We might reasonably aim to return the individual or system to precrisis level of functioning. The ultimate goal might be to improve the level of precrisis functioning to prevent future crises altogether or at least to manage them with improved efficiency. It is assumed that without support or intervention during the crisis period, an individual may never fully recover, which would result in less effective coping and negotiation of life in the future. With support and intervention, however, a crisis represents an opportunity for growth and change. Individuals can grow emotionally and become stronger following well-resolved crises.

Prevention Concepts and Mental Health Consultation

Another concept that has become a hallmark of prevention and crisis intervention is one frequently seen in the public health literature. This concept outlines various levels of the preventive process (Bloom, 1977; Caplan, 1964): primary prevention, secondary prevention, and tertiary prevention. Primary prevention includes activities that prevent crises from occurring altogether; secondary prevention includes activities that arrest potential crises from escalating; and tertiary prevention aims to repair damage from the occurrence of a crisis (i.e., crisis management). By way of illustration, then, primary prevention might consist of educating elementary school teachers about custody laws and establishing school policies and procedures to regulate authorized removal of children from the school. Effective implementation of such safeguards would constitute secondary prevention, and competent management of a crisis in which a child has been removed from school by an unauthorized person would be tertiary prevention.

School psychologists who have been trained in organizational and community intervention will quickly recognize primary and secondary prevention as the mainstay of most system-level intervention (Danish & D'Augelli, 1980; Rappaport, 1977; Reiff, 1975). To intervene at this level requires consultation skills. Consultation is a voluntary, nonsupervisory relationship between professionals from differing fields established to aid one in his or her professional functioning. What is the most effective way to work or consult with individuals in community agencies who know a great deal about their own institution but who perhaps have less of a background in mental health skills? Caplan (1970) outlined the basic components of this model in his book *The Theory and Practice of Mental Health Consultation.* These methodologies have been expanded and adapted for mental health professionals working in schools by several authors (see, for example, Conoley & Conoley, 1982; Gallessick, 1982).

In crisis intervention itself, the school psychologist might work directly with each particular case. However, the caseload would almost assuredly extend far beyond what is realistic for any district to support. An alternative, of course is to focus on establishing crisis intervention policies, procedures, and training programs throughout the school district in order to catch problems earlier and possibly to prevent them.

Kinds of Crisis

Several crisis theorists have attempted to develop categorical systems in attempts to generally classify various kinds of crises. Caplan (1964) discussed developmental crises (based on Erickson's work) as contrasted with situational crises (crises spawned by trauma). A more expanded taxonomy of crises was developed by Baldwin (1978) based on his work at a mental health clinic at the University of North Carolina. It delineates six major classifications of events associated with emotional crisis:

1. *Dispositional Crises.* The individual experiencing dispositional crises is primarily in need of information or reassurance to go about solving the problem he or she is confronted with. Baldwin (1978) describes the situation and the role of the intervener in this crisis as "distress resulting from a problematic situation in which the therapist responds to the client in ways peripheral to a therapeutic role; the intervention is not primarily directed at the emotional level" (p. 540).

2. *Anticipated Life Transitions.* Changes in life style that are reflective of essentially normal and anticipated progression make up this category, such as beginning/completing school, the birth of a sibling, or moving.

3. *Maturational/Developmental Crises.* These crises have to do with attempts to solve major life issues involving interpersonal problems. Such struggles include those revolving around sexual identity, dependency, of development or emotional intimacy.

4. *Traumatic Stress.* This results from unpredictable and uncontrollable stressors such as loss through death or divorce, physical abuse, or a series of traumatic events occurring rapidly together. This classification is probably the most typical crisis situation in schools today.

5. *Crises Reflecting Psychopathology.* These crises involve "a preexisting

psychopathology [that] has been instrumental in precipitating the crisis or in which psychopathology significantly impairs or complicates adaptive resolution" (Baldwin, 1978, p. 546). This category of crisis is seen much more often in school than in years past for reasons reviewed earlier. It appears that those working in the schools are likely to become accustomed to managing these more bizarre crises.

6. *Psychiatric Emergencies.* Those include "crisis situations in which general functioning has been severely impaired and the individual rendered incompetent or unable to assume personal responsibility" (p. 547). In these cases individuals may meet the "dangerous to self or others" standard for involuntary psychiatric evaluation and possible commitment. Increasingly, school psychologists are involved in or consulted regarding mental illness warrants for adult students or family members of students. Again, this is a fairly recent development and requires a knowledge of community resources and of the mental health judicial system preciding over the school district.

Most time and attention regarding crisis in the psychological and educational literature apply directly to individual crises in the lives of individual students and their families. However, to a greater or lesser extent, these events never occur on an individual basis. They can affect other children, the teacher, the counselor, the school, and the community. A shocking or traumatic event can potentially spark crises in large numbers of individuals. The effect such an event has on the school, together with the school system's attempts to negotiate or cope with it, is much more rarely examined. That such effects go unmeasured does not mean they are not staggering. When a child dies, for example, the entire school is affected in reviewing the issues revolving around loss and comprehension of death and of one's own mortality.

Often, however, the incident will be completely swept under the carpet, leaving faculty and students to wonder and seek out rumors. In these circumstances, it is hoped that questions arise regarding what should be told to other students, their parents, and the school staff as well as regarding how the staff should acknowledge or observe the crisis event. The school and community experience (to a varying extent depending on closeness to the deceased, etc.) many of the same issues that the child's family experiences. Crises in many ways can have an impact on an entire school community as well as on the individual involved. Some events typically pass with relatively little knowledge and therefore relatively little impact on the overall school environment. On the other hand, an incident as minor as a physically or emotionally out-of-control child can carry with it quite a pervasive impact on the school environment. An incident as major as a violent crime or accident with multiple deaths can result in emotional trauma in children and adults alike. However, the schools rarely are prepared to handle such conditions, which can perpetuate the same emotional reactions in groups of people as in individuals.

Thus, the theory and techniques employed when one is working with an individual in crisis frequently may need to be expanded to techniques needed for working with groups of individuals or organizations in crisis. Intervention in an organization or building full of individuals potentially in crisis requires all the skills necessary to address individual crisis management and a great number besides that are oriented toward management of the overall organizational upheaval. History, models, and techniques for this sort of intervention in the schools are reviewed in the final portion of this chapter.

SCHOOL PSYCHOLOGY IN CRISIS INTERVENTION

Theoretical considerations in the organizational/school crisis areas are based on many of the same concepts of community and consulting psychology. In fact, one could argue that some consulting and preventive aspects of the role of the school psychologist have evolved directly from early formulations and techniques of crisis intervention.

Interestingly, there is not a lot of attention in the literature given to school psychologists' involvement in crisis intervention prior to the 1980s. Certainly this may be a result of terminology (Wise & Smead, 1989). Our concept of "crisis intervention" skills may be referred to as "mental health consultation" (Meyers, 1981), "short-term dynamic therapies" (Barbanel, 1982), or be included under methods for attendance for specific crises such as divorce, suicide intervention, or grief counseling. However, even as recently as 1985, Smead noted that "to date there appear to be few reports of school psychologists using these (crisis intervention) approaches." This lack exists in spite of the fact that the potential for the application of preventive mental health services in general and crisis intervention specifically is tremendous and quite widely recognized (Nelson & Slaikeu, 1984). In fact, an informal scanning of the references for this book suggests that many of the school applications of crisis intervention are published in journals other than school psychology journals. Since 1985, only 11 articles using the terms crisis or crisis intervention have appeared in the *School Psychology Review* and the *Journal of School Psychology*.

Crisis as Opportunity

It is traditional and perhaps even a cliché by now to refer to the balance of danger and opportunity inherent in a crisis situation (see, for example, Wilheim, 1967; Lidell & Scott, 1968; Slaikeu, 1984). Perhaps this concept can be applied even at an organizational level. There is a very significant danger/opportunity aspect of crisis that we must understand and prepare ourselves and our profession to utilize. During and just subsequent to crisis there generally is thought to be reduced defensiveness or increased openness on the part of the system, again paralleling personal crisis.

Crisis frequently has opened the eyes of administrators and the community at large to the unmet mental health needs among children and adolescents. During crisis, these needs rise to a point where they can no longer be ignored. Once this awareness is established, perhaps accompanied by the significant motivation to avoid such an experience in the future, the school and community at large are generally more open to the necessary preventive measures that "helping" professions had been so urgently calling for. This process can, of course, happen much more efficiently if we as mental health professionals (1) recognize this opportunity and (2) are prepared to follow through with recommendatiaons and support necessary to guide schools and community agencies in a preventive direction.

2

Crisis in the Schools: Multiple Demands, Multiple Skills

GENERAL CONCEPTS AND INFORMATION

This chapter is divided between the skills involved with direct intervention in an "individual" crisis and those involved with consultation with school staff regarding their own management of crisis and its effects on their students.

Individual versus Organizational/Community Crises

Most time and attention regarding crisis in the psychological and educational literature apply directly to individual crises in the lives of "individual" students and their families. However, to a greater or lesser extent these events never occur on an individual basis. They affect other children, the teacher, the counselor, the school, and the greater community. The effects these events have even within the school are rarely examined as intensively as are the school system's attempts to negotiate or cope with them.

That such effects often go unnoticed does not mean they are not staggering. For a long time following a violent assault, neither children nor adults can walk into the building without a sense of vulnerability and perhaps even dread.

When a child dies, for example, the entire school is affected in reviewing the issues revolving around loss, comprehension of death, and of one's own mortality. As often as not the incident will be completely swept under the carpet, leaving faculty and students to wonder and seek out rumors. Ideally, however, questions will arise regarding what should be told to other students, their parents, the school staff, and how the staff should acknowledge or observe this event. The school and community experience (to a varying extent depending on closeness to the deceased) many of the same issues that the child's family experiences. However, school personnel rarely are prepared to handle such conditions; they can perpetuate the same emotional reactions in groups of people as in individuals. Thus, the theory and techniques employed when one is working with an individual in crisis frequently parallel those used in working with groups of individuals or organizations in crisis.

In many ways, crises fall on a continuum to the extent that they can affect an entire school community or only the individual involved. Some kinds of events typically pass with relatively little knowledge and therefore have little impact on the school. Others, even as much as a physically or emotionally out-of-control child, have seriously underestimated impacts.

Our intervention with crises must take this into account. In some cases, direct intervention with a child or adolescent is appropriate. In other instances, consultation with the administrative and teacher staff is best included. Furthermore, the school psychologist may be the individual to bring the need for building-level intervention to the administrator's attention. For example, Poland (1989a) described the teacher who insisted that her science students take an examination during the same class period that they heard about the suicide of their classmate. Through intervention of the school psychologist, the teacher was not allowed to give the test and was gently reminded that her methods were probably an attempt to manage her own emotions through denial of the event. At times, even intervention at the level of the school board or superintendent level may be necessary.

Crisis Intervention Is Interdisciplinary

In schools all professionals and paraprofessionals are faced with crisis situations. Teachers are certainly the front line in facing crises. Veteran teachers can usually relate a number of shocking crisis situations they have confronted. This dynamic does not stop with teachers. Ask the bus drivers, the secretaries, and the janitors. They too have stories regarding serious crises confided to them or otherwise "dropped" on them by students. One teacher from a small town in the midwest shared a story about the student who threatened suicide because she was pregnant after a relationship with the high school coach. Recently in our experience, a junior high student arrived at school for his first class and announced to his teacher that he had shot both of his parents that morning.

Crisis intervention skills are for all school personnel. Every one who faces crises should be trained to manage them as far as is appropriate to his or her role. Frequently mental health professionals are most aware of the need for crisis skills and planning and consider skills to be within their professional role only. This exclusivity is unwarranted and unrealistic. We must remember that for one reason or another most crises are managed without the intervention of a mental health professional. One recent study suggested that teachers most frequently consulted another teacher or their school principal regarding what to do about a crisis situation (Wise & Smead, 1989).

Even most mental health professionals do not have crisis intervention training or field experience. Knowledge of psychopathology, learning theory, and personality dynamics may be helpful but is no substitute for the skill of lethality assessment or the ability to convene community resources rapidly. The American Association of Suicidology recommends a minimum of 40 hours of crisis training as their standard program (American Association of Suicidology, 1976a,b). Therefore, school districts might consider sending individuals who manage crises to in-service training programs conducted in the community.

A CONCEPTUAL MODEL OF CRISIS

In an attempt to sort out a general understanding of what crisis is, it is helpful to think of an event and the reaction to it as occurring in three phases (Golan, 1978). The crisis model delineated applies to personal crises among students as well as to staff reactions. A different set of intervention objectives and activities are associated with each phase. These phases and activities are outlined in Table 2.1.

The Impact Phase

Often during a crisis, or what is experienced as a crisis by staff, emotions run high, and a simple logical solution is easy to overlook. For this reason it can be helpful to keep in mind this simple model for intervening in the impact phase (Leviton & Greenstone, 1989). We have found it

TABLE 2.1. Phases of Crisis Intervention

1. Impact phase	Primary prevention activities
2. Recoil stage	Secondary prevention activities
3. Resolution or adjustment phase	Secondary prevention activities
4. Return to precrisis functioning level	Tertiary prevention activities

convenient and flexibly applicable in an educational setting. This model summarizes primary prevention steps:

1. Immediately take steps to gain control.
2. Once a crisis is under control, take some time to quickly assess the situation.
3. Make dispositions and decisions; impose consequences for inappropriate behavior.
4. Make referrals and follow-up; review management system and come up with a realistic plan for how such situations can be managed in the future.

In a large, suburban school district, policy changes prompted administrators to educate some behaviorally disordered, mentally retarded students in the district facility rather than to send these students to residential settings. Shortly thereafter the author was asked to come to the campus because Tommy, a rather large and menacing mentally retarded, autistic young man, had left his classroom and was going from classroom to classroom punching teachers. The staff and director had previously experienced very compliant students who responded to a firm voice. To them this sort of threatening behavior was quite terrorizing.

According to the model of intervention, control was the first goal. Physically overpowering this young man was out of the question and probably not necessary. Each teacher was simply asked to close his or her door (locked from the inside). The first goal of ensuring the safety of students and staff was thus very simply met. Next, security was called, and four adults gave Tommy a choice of going to the "quiet room" or having his mother called and going home. Tommy chose the quiet room and worked for the balance of the day in this isolated setting. Thus, the immediate crisis was under control, and we were free to move on to the second phase.

"Getting control" is a skill in itself, and toward the end of this section of the book, it is examined in more depth. Suffice it to say at present that almost never is physical intervention on the part of the school psychologist or even other school personnel appropriate.

In this case, assessment involved gathering more information about Tommy and the staff. Had this sort of thing occurred before? What management techniques had been attempted and failed? His parents were contacted to apprise them of the situation and to obtain further input.

A plan was then formulated for how to handle Tommy after he left the designated area. A brief staff meeting was held before teachers left for the day to provide for ventilation and to develop a temporary contingency plan for the following day.

We have here a fairly simple situation with a fairly simple solution, right? Let's take just a moment, though, to consider how this seemingly simple crisis situation could have escalated. What if the intervener immediately proceeded to "make" Tommy return to class. What if the intervener squared off with Tommy and with a raised voice stated "Tommy, get back to class"? Tommy continued to have control over the situation. If he chose to follow the directive, fine. If he did not, he might well escalate and become more violent. In this later scenario, the situation has at best remained in the crisis state and might have become worse. Even in the event that Tommy responded to someone firm whom he might not have known so well, it was a gamble that might not pay off again in the future.

Recoil Phase

During the recoil phase, the immediate crisis has passed. The reactions of those experiencing the crisis are just beginning to "set in." Tearfulness, denial, and anger are all common emotional reactions during this phase. It is an immediate emotional and sometimes physical "backlash." Usually this is a time for individuals to be aware that it's productive to talk with each other about their reactions, that emotional and fearful reactions are "normal" for a shocking situation, and that, given time, they will adjust (i.e., these emotions will fade).

After the "Tommy" incident, teachers told us that they went home that night and cried from the shock of being attacked by one of their students. For some it was difficult to walk back into the building the following day. It was fairly simple to encourage some sharing of these reactions in this small building where the authors were well known. However, even after a simple and brief discussion, more severe stress generally was reduced to mere shaking of heads and dismissal.

Resolution or Adjustment Phase

During the resolution phase, individuals slowly get over the initial strong emotional recoil. This period takes much longer than the period where anxiety and emotionality shoots up (see Figure 2-1).

Once over the initial emotional recoil from the "Tommy" incident, staff were able to adjust to the long-term significance, or in some cases changes, that the crisis signaled. Later we had time to make a more thorough behavior modification plan with the staff. Although we would do everything possible to prevent it, the truth was that Tommy would stay at their school and might act out again. What's more, it looked as if the staff might be educating a more "crisis-prone" student in the future.

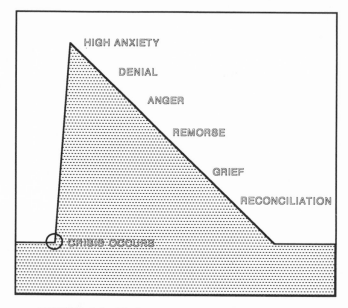

FIGURE 2.1. Victims response to emotional crisis.

Precrisis Functioning Level

After a period of time, most individuals adjust completely to the crisis event and the changes it may have brought. This is a slow process and takes from months to years. Some months later everyone was adjusted to Tommy's episodes of aggressive behavior. Several teachers took classes designed to help them in the management of violent student behavior; others eventually transferred to other educational settings in the district.

MANAGEMENT OF THE CRISIS CALL

If you have been working in the schools or other mental health agencies for very long, you will be familiar with this particular type of crisis phone call. The emotional content is very high. The range of incidents perceived as crises is extremely variable. It includes problems such as "come right away—we can't locate the proper referral form" to "a student just came to school and shot someone." Whatever the precipating incident, some basic elements are consistently included.

1. We have a problem we can't handle.
2. You must have a solution.
3. You should come here immediately and offer it.

Since these calls often appear to the psychologist to be a tempest in a teapot, there is a continuing temptation to avoid them, especially if he or she is a salaried employee of the school district and has many other responsibilities. It is only human to grow weary of frequent annoying calls, especially those that appear to be unrealistically panicky. Yet, it is also a grave necessity that news of serious situations be made known to you immediately. There are few circumstances that reduce credibility of a support person as quickly as not delivering on a promised or relied on role when the consultee is in crisis.

When possible, frequent, somewhat inappropriate crisis calls should be viewed as a signal for more training for the individuals involved. The crisis interventionist should remember that often the individuals placing the call are experiencing the same level of emotional turmoil we associate with more major upheavals. We can predict and plan for many situations in which frequent calls will occur. They are situations that involve any change in the existing school community: new programs are placed on a campus, a new school opens, or a new and unusual student is placed on a campus.

When calls must be prioritized, it can be very helpful as well as time efficient to rely on someone in your office to screen calls. All nonemergency contacts are recorded as messages and can be returned at the finish of the day. In this manner when you receive a call, you can be sure you need to act immediately. This simple policy can practically ensure that a significant problem will not be overlooked.

If it is unrealistic to believe that one crisis interventionist could always be available in the face of a serious crisis (and generally it is), then backups must be appointed. In the schools the hours of crisis are generally limited by the hours of the school day, so for many districts, the constant availability of *someone* is not an unrealistic expectation.

Informational Content of the Crisis Call

When the call does come in, it is important to learn as much as possible about the nature of a crisis before becoming involved (Zizzo, 1989). Begin intervention immediately by responding in a logical and calming manner. Below is a checklist of key questions that should be answered if you are to prepare to respond to the crisis effectively.

1. What happened, exactly?
2. Have other necessary professionals been called? (School social worker, the police, medical emergency personnel, school security, superintendent, etc. If not and they are necessary, they should be called immediately by someone at the scene.)
3. Have the necessary family or significant others been contacted?
4. Has the person been apprehended? Is the event still occurring?
5. How many people were affected? Where are they?
6. What is the extent of the damage? What is the current state of the building?

These questions apply equally well across most crisis situations from one in which a young child becomes violent in an elementary school to a more bizarre and unusual case of a natural disaster or a bus accident.

Questions You Should Ask Yourself

What resources will I need? One person is often not enough if a number of individuals at the school have been affected. What other resource individuals might be available to help out, and which of these individuals would be the most valuable? Sometimes materials are necessary such as suicide contracts, lists of local community resources, or other educational information for the individuals on the campus.

Who should be alerted before I go? Frequently others need to know where you are and what sort of crisis you are responding to. If you are leaving your regular services, the building will need to be briefly informed of the necessity of your departure.

After the crisis is managed, who needs to be contacted? What follow-up work needs to occur? A phone call to the parents, a check with your office, and/or a "debriefing" for school personnel involved or interested is often in order.

WHAT YOU NEED TO KNOW ABOUT YOUR COMMUNITY MENTAL HEALTH SYSTEM

One Friday afternoon a psychologist had been asked to manage a crisis situation by the school counselor. A senior had come to the counselor's office in a very distraught emotional state. She reported that she had been dating a young man of different ethnic background for several months and approximately 4 days earlier had told her father about it. Her father had violently objected to the relationship. He had not gone to work since he had received the news, staying home in bed most of the time. She proceeded to relate that the situation frightened her a great deal for historical reasons: her father was a recovering alcoholic, had attempted suicide and homicide previously, and had seen two mental health professionals (a psychologist and a church counselor), who had both recommended hospitalization. Further, he was threatening to kill her, the young man, and himself. There were a number of guns at his disposal. She was understandably very concerned and panicked at prospect of the upcoming weekend.

Resources included an older sister (22 years) and a mother who had a history of noninvolvement and refusal to exercise her rights to protect her family. All the known information suggested that this situation involved a very real life-and-death threat. How is a crisis worker to say to a near-hysterical adolescent girl, "Sorry, your hour is up" and leave for the weekend? Alternatively, what can the crisis worker personally do to resolve such a situation?

These situations are not rare. In our experience such legitimate "life-and-death" situations do arise; commonly they arise on Friday afternoons. The escalating potential crisis situation comes to a head when the individual is confronted with an upcoming weekend. It is not realistic to continue to work over weekends, nor are resolutions for such scenarios within our grasp. Crisis workers must be educated regarding other support help within the communities. What follows is a short list of community supports, agencies that crisis workers in the schools will need to rely on consistently.

Duty to Warn

We have all been schooled regarding the significance of confidentiality in a therapeutic relationship. However, there are clear limits to confidentiality. When a client is imminently homicidal or suicidal, it is mandatory that confidentiality be broken. What's more, the student should be aware that this is the case from the onset of any crisis counseling. Such crisis counselors go so far as to insist that students (especially conduct-disordered, personality-disordered individuals) sign a written statement of these policies at some appropriate point near the beginning of counseling.

For most school-aged individuals, the parents must be contacted; sometimes both parents and a juvenile parole officer need to be alerted. If the threat is against another person, that person or his or her parents must be contacted. There are no exceptions to this protocol.

Many times this dynamic does raise questions such as "will the student openly discuss such personal impulses if he or she is aware they will not go unreported?" We have found that this is not a major problem in the vast majority of cases. If handled with sensitivity and support, most students will, in the long run, understand that such methods are designed to help them.

Involuntary and Voluntary Commitment Processes

The need for knowledge regarding these processes often enters into crisis counseling either directly (the student may require psychiatric observation, most often in the case of imminent suicide) or indirectly (through a family member or friend). Each state and community observes a slightly different process, so crisis workers will need to educate themselves regarding their own community policies.

The standard of "dangerous to self or others" is quite uniformly. Usually a family member or neighbor will need to present clear verbal evidence to a judge that the individual in question is imminently dangerous—not just bizarre or unpredictable. For example, a man who lives across the street walking about the neighborhood at night screaming that he is receiving signals from his TV set that the world is ending would probably not qualify for mental illness arrest. If, however, this same man became annoyed at the neighbor's dog and broke a window threatening to "carve him up," the evidence would probably be seen as much more convincing.

The judge would then issue some form of order (in Texas it's a Mental Illness Warrant) for the individual to be arrested and brought to a psychiatric hospital for observation and recommendation. Sometimes the individuals are released after this observation period (usually about 48 hours), and sometimes they are involuntarily committed or hospitalized for a month or more.

Private Psychiatric Hospitalization and Psychiatrists

Many individuals will approach you with questions regarding possible private hospitalization or psychiatric assessment. A current list of recommended individuals and institutions should be kept on hand. This list should probably be comprised of professionals who have a proven track record and have shown consideration for family long-term need. For example, some psychiatric hospitals routinely exhaust lifetime mental health insurance benefits on the first treatment. We refer to those hospitals that attempt to balance services for the client's long-term benefit, for example, those that manage treatment so that the client has some benefits left for additional treatment after leaving the hospital, those that hospitalize only when no alternative exists, etc.

It is often beneficial to visit hospitals and discuss these policies openly with them. Some sort of routine interaction with community mental health professionals, such as biannual professional luncheons, also provides a simple vehicle to "catch up with the latest" developmental advances in private human service personnel.

Emergency Family Counseling Resources

Many hospitals and community clinics offer emergency counseling services that can involve the entire family. Some communities offer these services on a 24-hour basis. Lists of such services will probably need to include alternatives that are private (and usually quite costly) and lists of agencies that can deliver services based on ability to pay. In the majority of these referral instances, financial circumstances will preclude full private fees.

Telephone Crisis Facilities

We recommend that the crisis worker carry cards printed with telephone crisis lines (if they are available in your community). Crises will occur on weekends and evenings, and school-based crisis personnel cannot take responsibility for these periods. Giving out the home telephone number not only paves the road to burnout but is also misleading to the client. The crisis worker will not always be available. If this is the only number the client is armed with, and the crisis worker cannot be reached, it will at least undermine the relationship and at worst initiate some sort of panic triggering a maladaptive response in the client (suicide attempt, running away from home, etc.).

Child Protection Agencies and Policies

The crisis worker will need to be aware of how and when to report child abuse and what to expect from the child protective agencies. In most communities such agencies are wildly understaffed and therefore limited. These limitations should be clearly defined in advance for the crisis worker. Many times children will not be removed from what appears to be an obviously dangerous situation. Crisis workers must understand the legal limitations and removal policies. On occasion crisis workers will be threatened by parents who are upset about such a report. Some advance thought and mental preparation should also be given to the possibilities of such an occurrence.

Juvenile Justice System and Policies

Students involved in crisis often have a police record or are committing offenses in violation of the law. Local agencies are usually very willing to educate crisis workers regarding when to report behaviors, what incarceration policies are, etc.

CRISIS COUNSELING SKILLS AND METHODS

There are many treatment strategies presented in the crisis literature. Because a number of studies have suggested generic patterns of response to stressful situations (Bowlby, 1960; Janis, 1958; Kaplan & Mason, 1960; Lindemann, 1944; Rapoport, 1963; Tyhurst, 1957), most of the treatment strategies focus on a particular crisis (e.g., bereavement, rape, or death of a loved one) rather than on the intrapsychic world of each individual. For this reason, crisis counseling is especially suited to groups aimed at commonalities of crisis experience (Jacobson, Strickler, & Morely, 1968).

Response to crisis in general has been recognized by other theorists (Bowlby, 1960; Dixon, 1979; Golan, 1978; Janis, 1958; Kaplan & Mason, 1960; Lindemann, 1944; Rapoport, 1963; Tyhurst, 1957) as being uniform enough to present a more general framework of crisis intervention practice that can be utilized regardless of what the crisis may be. Overall, activities usually include tension reduction through emotional and physical catharsis, encouragement of interpersonal interaction for social support, direct encouragement of adaptive behavior, and provision of coping and mastery experience and environmental manipulation.

Why School-Based Crisis Therapy?

It becomes very difficult to ignore crisis counseling or maintain that it is outside the domain of education when students come to school unable to learn and, at times, too tearful or panic-stricken to remain in class without embarrassment and extreme discomfort on the part of other students and teachers. Sometimes these events may occur during the school day within the building: a student or teacher dies, or an accident occurs involving many injuries. Most commonly, however, students bring with them the aftermath of tragic events and circumstances in the home and community: a car accident kills a number of peers, sexual and physical abuse is revealed, a suicide of a friend or family member occurs, or parents divorce.

As summarized in Chapter 1, research and clinical experience overwhelmingly suggest that crises and extreme stress during childhood adversely affect performance, behavior, and overall adjustment (Cowen & Hightower, 1986). Traditionally educators and mental health professionals have waited for stressed children to find their way to "repair" services in the formal health services delivery system. Realistically, we know that many do not. Instead they continue to struggle with negative psychological consequences long after. Resources should be available to provide temporary, general crisis intervention support in the environment that the child must negotiate every day.

Goals of Crisis Therapy

Crisis intervention is very different from psychotherapy. A crisis is not the time to delve into an individual's personality or long-term problems unrelated to the crisis. If and when these personality issues arise in the course of working toward crisis resolution, the crisis worker knows that such issues are not the domain of crisis work. He or she acknowledges the existence of the issue and recommends a psychotherapy or another counseling resource.

Common Therapeutic Issues and Themes among Children

Psychotherapeutic issues that appear to be generically related to those experiencing crisis include those discussed in the following paragraphs.

Distrust

This phenomenon appears to be especially present in older children or adolescents who have been chronically exposed to an ongoing extreme stressor or for whom a good deal of time has elapsed since the crisis event or events. The natural and adaptive attitude is to increase defensiveness and develop strong guards against intimacy. Even though rapport is well established at the onset of therapy, continuing issues surrounding trust will probably continue to emerge. Probably the most consistent, long-standing challenge for individuals who have experienced severe crises in their lives is the establishment of intimate relationships.

Guilt

This emotion surfaces again and again throughout all sorts of crisis experiences. Sources of guilt are usually quite irrational. The most common include (1) blaming oneself for the occurrence of the crisis event (common in children experiencing divorce and death), (2) feeling "unworthy" of surviving a crisis that others did not, and (3) actions that the individual regrets ("I could have done more; I never should have . . .").

There is some evidence to indicate that if therapeutic intervention is still ongoing long after an extremely stressful event (e.g., the holocaust), the crisis trauma may be a nearly unalterable pattern (Chodoff, 1980). It is hoped, although not empirically established, that therapeutic intervention soon after the crisis event(s) may help prevent such long-standing negative emotions.

Control

Many times children attempt to solve crisis-related problems that are beyond their control. This may be a reaction to the helplessness of being "victimized" by the crisis. An important aspect in therapy is often to help patients first to distinguish the problems that are beyond their control and to activate any problem-solving strategies only when problems are within patient control.

Anger and Revenge

This reaction can be directed at the perceived instigator of the crisis or at the caretaker for not protecting the child adequately. Identification with the aggressor is also a pattern that appears at times. The child may model him- or herself after the perceived perpetrator of the crisis.

Avoidance

Often there is avoidance of people, places, and experiences that the child fears because of their key role in the crisis. This avoidance can become generalized and negatively affect the adjustment of the child in a variety of similar experiences. As soon as a child has recuperated from the initial shock, a successive approximations approach may be used to gradually reduce and eliminate this phenomenon.

Therapist Reactions

It can be difficult to work with children and adolescents who have experienced some rather horrific incidents. Such reactions can interfere with empathy and understanding as well as the firmness and consistency that are necessary to work with children. It can be tempting to feel a bit guilty oneself if one's own children or childhood was happy, supportive, and healthy.

A Generic Crisis Counseling Model

No matter what particular characteristics are included in the crisis incident, certain phases or steps in therapy have been classically cited in the literature (Morley, Messick, & Aguilera, 1967). This generic approach is based on the concept of the therapist as problem solver, that is, facilitator of a rational sorting out of the problems and options for an individual who has temporarily lost this capacity because of overwhelming emotional interference: anxiety, anger, sorrow.

One specific approach, The Life Space Interviewing Approach (developed in the late 1960s by Redl, 1969), was specifically developed to assist professionals working with children who were very upset. The overall approach can be broken down into a general sequence of techniques: listening or information-gathering phase, gathering information pertaining to frequency and duration of the problem, gathering specific details of what happened, and providing support for the child through the use of active listening skills. We have included techniques described in crisis literature (adapted to relate to children and adolescents in an educational environment) together with Redl's Life Space Interviewing and suggest the following general approach. These phases follow an order, although they may vary in the amount of time spent in each one.

Assessment

The first task is to identify, define, and focus the problem. During this phase the therapist attempts to gain an understanding of the event that precipitated the crisis and the student's interpretation of the crisis situation. The entire assessment process amounts to a careful search for information to help the therapist form a picture of the individual's situation from both a subjective and an objective viewpoint. A picture of the individual's thoughts and feelings slowly emerges, and frequently this exercise in itself is therapeutic and to some extent cathartic. Information important to gain during this phase is the specific definition of the problem. The successful formulation of a plan to cope will depend on the information produced by this careful assessment phase. Pertinent questions during the assessment phase include:

- What happened? (Identify the precipitating event. It could be anything: physical or sexual abuse, parental fight or divorce, loss of boyfriend or girlfriend, or unwanted pregnancy, to list a few.)
- When did it happen? (The precipitating event usually occurs within 10 to 14 days before the individual seeks counseling.)
- Why at this point has the individual sought out counseling attention?

- What does this event mean to him or her? How does the individual perceive the event in the present, and what effect does he or she feel it will have on him or her in the future? (A determination is made of how realistic or distorted the individual's interpretations of the situation are.)
- What situational supports are available? Does the individual have someone close to talk with. Who is his or her best friend? Is there someone in his or her family who is loved and trusted? Is there someone he or she can talk with outside of the school environment?
- Does this individual have a history of strong coping skills? Has anything like this ever happened before? What methods have worked in the past to cope with fear, sadness, anger? What would help to reduce the negative emotions now felt?
- How much has the crisis interrupted the individual's life? Is the individual still able to go to or function in school or work? Is the individual able to locate somewhere safe to live? How is the incident affecting those around him or her: parents, other family members, siblings, etc.? What have significant others advised him or her to do?
- A careful assessment should be made for suicidal and homicidal potential. Should specific and direct questions be asked (see Poland, 1989a, for detailed approaches)? Has the person developed any plans to the point of having a realistic method readily available? How many details have been thought out? (Of course, if some suggestion is present regarding a potential for suicide, a referral should be made for private, more prolonged, and intensive treatment, possibly in a hospital. It is important to gain an understanding of how much the crisis has disrupted the individual's day-to-day functioning; for example, have attendance, peer relationships, family relationships, activity level, academic performance been affected?)

The therapist should be listening for (adapted from *Field Manual for Human Service Workers in Major Disasters,* NIMH, 1978):

- Concern about basic survival potential for suicide or fears regarding physical safety.
- Grief over loss of loved ones, status, possessions.
- Separation anxiety that can be expressed as fears regarding the safety of loved ones or that center directly on the person involved.
- Regressive behaviors, such as increased attachment to blankets, stuffed animals, thumb sucking, clinginess, etc.
- Anxiety regarding possible relocation or isolation because of the crisis event.

Therapeutic Intervention—Child or Adolescent

Throughout the assessment phase the therapist remains alert for strengths of the individual and discusses coping strategies and supports that are available to the individual and have been attempted or are available but are not in use. With children, some version of this discussion often must occur with parents at a later time.

During therapeutic intervention, an attempt is made to identify each potential option the individual has at that time. A severe crisis often causes disorganization in thinking and functioning. One reaction to the crisis situation is a feeling of being overwhelmed and an inability to act. It is helpful to select one most immediate problem (if many are identified) and focus on it first. If a problem can be identified that is readily solvable, the resulting success will be important in bringing back a sense of control and a feeling of confidence.

Intervention

The particular intervention techniques will depend heavily on the nature of the child's problem, his family situation, and the skills and creativity of the therapist. Overall, then, the therapist defines the problem and summarizes all the pertinent information for the crisis person. The two then move into exploring possible alternative solutions for the individual. Each option is discussed with an understanding of its probable positive and negative consequences.

Morley suggests a number of approaches that may be wedded with the information presented above regarding possible problems that may be present because of crisis. Morley's suggestions include:

- Helping the student realistically to evaluate his or her situation cognitively and emotionally.
- Helping the student recognize emotional reactions that are present but that he or she does not fully recognize or acknowledge.
- Exploring alternative methods of coping or looking at the situation.
- Expanding the social world (involving others for social support).

Further techniques that can be useful with children and adolescents include:

- Assuring the student that strong emotional reactions and many of his or her own emotions are normal for individuals experiencing this particular crisis.

- Helping the individual to gain an intellectual understanding of his or her emotional experiences (e.g., stages in grief, time-relatedness of grief symptoms).
- Establishing realistic goals for the near future.

At the end of this discussion, however, the individual must leave with a specific agreed-on plan or initial solution. An aim should be made to keep the student involved in construction of the plan, which should encourage a sense of power and hasten the point in time when the individual might resume his or her own independent functioning. If necessary a plan for even one day at a time is constructed. Also a specific time in the near future should be designated for a meeting during which to monitor the effectiveness of the attempted solutions and to reformulate them if necessary.

Resolution

This phase occurs during follow-up meeting(s) and includes encouraging those coping mechanisms that are constructive and seem to be serving the individual well. Progress in understanding should be noted and praised, and one should anticipate that the individual may feel some embarrassment in future encounters at school when he or she is feeling better. Most importantly, promises should not be made for services or materials or solutions that may not be available. Never promise:

- Not to disclose information under any circumstances, especially those in which danger to self or others is implicated.
- To be available to the individual outside of work hours.
- To support action from another agency that has not been fully confirmed.

Toward the end of the first session, it helps to remind children that all information will be kept confidential. They needn't worry whether their parents or teachers will "know" unless they so desire. Attempt to "normalize" the crisis counseling process by noting that, although everyone has very personal and unique problems, many students have times in their lives when their problems seem overwhelming.

Frequently the resolution phase does not receive real closure for the therapist. Once the individual feels better, especially if the individual is an adolescent, he or she may attempt to cope with the crisis to some extent by denying it. It may therefore be embarrassing or stressful to the individual to acknowledge the conversation or crisis in the future, and some sensitivity and understanding should be shown on the part of the therapist.

Counseling for Anxiety: Stress Inoculation Treatment

One of the most frequent emotional childhood reactions to crisis is fear. Temporary irrational fears emerge that the child has great difficulty managing. One model for intervention with such fears was originally proposed by Meichenbaum (1975) and advocated since it was useful with postdisaster fear reactions in children (Auerbach & Spirito, 1986). The approach essentially teaches children to change their internal cognitive interpretations and "self-talk" and allows them little by little to de-sensitize themselves to the fear.

Meichenbaum's approach consists of three distinct phases. During the first, the primary focus is on education. During this phase the child's experience is "normalized," and he or she is told that it is not unusual to have this reaction. The child is then encouraged to describe in detail what his or her thoughts, feelings, and interpretations were during the incident. The therapist then notes these internal dialogues for future work.

During the second phase, the "rehearsal phase," a number of techniques might be employed. Relaxation-training techniques can be particularly helpful in reducing anxiety, including the children's version of the traditional deep muscle relaxation training (Koeppen, 1974), which involves fantasy. Imagery-involved techniques might also help the children to experience physical relaxation while mentally (or sometimes physically) confronting the feared stimulus or event.

Another group of techniques that might be implemented during the rehearsal phase involve changing the child's "self-talk," which should result eventually in behavioral change (Meichenbauam, 1977). Training programs that focus specifically on helping children to use these techniques include Spirito and Finch (1980) and Kendall and Braswell (1984). Meichenbaum and Goodman (1971) describe the steps involved:

1. Cognitive modeling—therapist talks aloud to him- or herself, modeling the task for the child.
2. Overt, external guidance—the child is asked to perform a given task while verbally guiding him- or herself out loud.
3. Faded overt self-guidance—the child performs the same task while whispering to him- or herself instead of talking out loud.
4. Covert self-instruction—the child performs the task while talking to him- or herself silently or "in his or her head."

A primary emphasis for such "thought replacement" is the negative interpretations or thoughts involving the crisis or disaster. If the child will volunteer or can clearly articulate the thoughts that are producing anxiety, he or she can then replace them with "coping" positive thoughts that presumably cause much less anxiety. Four general types of verbalizations are modeled for the child: (a) problem definition (What is the best thing to do?); (2) focusing of attention (I must look carefully and take my time); (3) coping statements (Something scared me at school yesterday, but today it is safe); or (4) self-rewarding (I am handling this well, even though I still feel a little frightened). When these are applied in the context of crisis intervention, probably more focus will be placed on coping and self-rewarding statements than on other more traditional applications of such procedures (e.g., children with attentional problems).

The third phase or "application phase" is the time to test the newly developed coping skills. The child attempts to confront an anxiety-producing situation little by little if necessary and manage his or her fear.

One feature of this program that lends it to widespread applicability for children in schools is that it can be conducted in classrooms by teachers for large groups of children. Although there has been no systematic evaluation of the procedure vis-à-vis crisis, common sense dictates that the group support aspect, so commonly found to be a key in improved functioning, would strengthen the cognitive procedures.

Counseling for Loss, Death, and Mourning

Many crises that surface in the school environment involve grief over tragic events. In fact, in the crisis literature, "crisis intervention" refers solely to crisis counseling/therapeutic skills. An example of the first type of treatment strategy is the model presented by Lindemann (1944) for the crisis of bereavement. In this model, Lindemann lists a number of psychological tasks that patients must complete if they are to successfully resolve the death of a loved one. The list of tasks is basically the same for every individual whether male or female, rich or poor, and comprises what is referred to as a "generic approach." This list of psychological tasks that the therapist helps the individual complete during the course of treatment includes:

1. Accept the pain of bereavement.
2. Review his relationship with the deceased and become acquainted with the alterations in his/her own modes of emotional reaction.
3. Express sorrow and a sense of loss.
4. Find an acceptable formulation of his/her future relationship to the deceased.
5. Verbalize his/her feelings of guilt and find persons around him

whom he can use as "primers" for acquisition of new patterns of conduct. (Lindemann, 1944, p. 147)

It is not unusual for the death, divorce, or loss of an individual in a child's life to trigger questions about death and dying. The fear of the loss and divorce of their own parents underlies many of these questions. When a mother or father dies, most children are fearful of losing the other parent as well. Being told that they will be taken care of is reassuring. As with other crisis situations, the children should be encouraged to voice their questions, and the adult should do the best he or she can to answer the questions honestly, for example, "the wisest men and women through the ages have tried to answer this question, but there is no sure answer." Explanations alluding briefly to heaven or hell, afterlife, or saying that after death there is "nothing" can create more anxiety for the child.

Many times a child must be reminded that adults around him or her also are feeling emotional pain and managing it in their own way. It can be very frightening to a child to suddenly experience crying or angry outbursts in adults who never before acted this way. Acknowledgment of the death and discussions about feelings, wishes, fears, etc., are very important for the child's adjustment. Generally, strongly emotional reactions (extreme crying, angry pounding of fists) should be expressed in the company of other adults. On the other end of the continuum, it is also very confusing to children to observe no reaction at all in important figures in their lives.

Frequently children may make believe that the lost parent is alive. Questions such as "When will Daddy wake up from being dead?" or wavering back and forth in believing that the parent actually died are not uncommon. Since denial of the death is frequently prevalent in children, they may become angry when challenged or told that the deceased parent will not return.

Because children engage in magical thinking or believe that their fantasies might influence reality, they may need to be reassured that prior angry thoughts or wishes did not cause the death to occur. One example that surfaces quite commonly is that a child may believe that fighting with his or her brother caused the death to occur and that if he or she resists fighting it will prevent the death of other significant others in his life. It is comforting to remind the child that these are things he or she cannot control. It can be contrasted with things that the child can control, such as doing homework, assigned household tasks, or playing fairly in a game.

Losses of pets or sentimental objects can have as much effect on children as the loss of a loved one. Children going through crisis or disaster often retrieve objects that appear to be of little rational use. However, these can be a reminder of security and involve great sentiment to the child at the time and should be recognized as important.

It is important for anyone working with children experiencing mourning to be aware that it is important for both children and their parents to cry. It is usually necessary to remind the child that thoughts about the loved one will come back again and again for a while and that the adjustment will take time. The family and teachers need to develop patience and supportive attitudes with the child who asks the same questions about death and loss again and again. They need to be aware that this is the child's way of adapting to the loss.

Mourning, the adaptation to loss, has been seen as involving the four basic tasks outlined below. It is essential that the grieving person accomplish these tasks before mourning can be completed. Uncompleted grief tasks can impair further growth and development. Although the tasks do not necessarily follow a specific order, there is some ordering suggested in the definitions. If grief were compared to physical healing (Engel, 1961), it is possible for someone to accomplish some of these tasks and not others and end up with what he calls an "incomplete" bereavement, just as one might have incomplete healing from a wound. The four tasks of mourning are as follows, according to Worden (1982):

1. To accept the reality of the loss. Denying the facts of loss can vary in degree from a slight distortion to a full-blown delusion. Typically someone will go through "mummification" of the individual's things or possessions. Another self-protection device is to deny the meaning of the loss.
2. To experience the pain of grief.
3. To adjust to an environment in which the deceased is missing.
4. To withdraw emotional energy and reinvest it in another relationship.

Group Counseling

The opportunity to work one-to-one with students or faculty is often simply not a realistic option. When caught in a similar situation in the 1940s, Veterans Administration hospital staff piloted the use of treatment groups, and a large body of literature has since evolved regarding group counseling techniques. Group counseling sessions can often not only prove economical but be the treatment of choice for many crisis situations. Group support has been shown to be very effective with children and adolescents for a number of crisis-related therapies (Cowen & Hightower, 1986). We have already noted that human beings experience crisis in fairly predictable ways. We have also noted the goals for therapy, especially if the individuals are all reacting to the same crisis event, as they frequently are in the schools (i.e., death/suicide of peer). The group experience for children of latency age and older seems more natural to them because of their daily routine in classroom settings. Especially at the adolescent level, irrational beliefs and behavior that an individual cannot recognize in himself or in herself may be recognized in peers.

A second aspect of crisis counseling that lends itself to group thera-peutic approaches is that crisis counseling, in theory and technique, assumes that there is no individual pathology per se. It presupposes that a series of shock reactions, if you will, are perfectly normal for any individual experiencing a shock or crisis. Crisis counseling is, therefore, only a method to guide people through the natural healing process with support and possibly some redirection of any irrational, destructive ideology. The process of working with a mental health professional together in a group with those experiencing the same shock or crisis is far less stigmatizing than going by oneself to see the "doctor." This is especially so, since many individuals in this process may tend to "blame themselves" or feel guilty in some way for the crisis event.

If groups are to be used, children should probably be grouped accord-ing to their age and level of exposure to the event/level of stress. A social support system provided by past and future association (neighborhood, class) tends to alleviate effects of various sorts of stress and helps the individual to cope with stress (Caplan, 1974; Cobbs, 1976). A group treatment format of short-term, crisis-oriented broad-spectrum group counseling is optimal.

Generally group treatment for crisis intervention purposes consists of small groups of students (about five to eight in number). Students selected for group should be emotionally balanced and willing to partici-pate in the group. Assignment to a group should follow the natural social support system as much as possible (i.e., neighborhood, home-room, etc.). Frequently it is helpful to space sessions much closer together (approximately one per day for a few days, the one per week) just following the crisis, with the last few separated by longer periods, such as a few weeks. Most professionals report that the most intense upset following a crisis is overcome in 1 to 6 weeks. Scheduling group sessions to roughly coincide with this time period should cover most "normal" disaster or community crisis situations.

Social support should be modeled and otherwise encouraged. Groups function best when the leaders are democratic and care about the mem-bers. The authoritarian manner discourages the use of free discussion, and students avoid speaking about fears, anxieties, etc.

Several excellent group formats have been developed for children experiencing various sorts of trauma. In general, these programs include activities such as role playing, skits, and filmstrips that generate discussion on (1) creating a protective setting to vent and express feelings and fears (usually these fears include loss of control over one's life or environment and unpredictability of what the future may hold; group leaders model empathy, respect, warmth, genuineness); (2) the relationship between the crisis event and feelings; (3) replacing irrational fears with realistic assessments of the situation and coping statements; (4) ways that strong emotions can affect behavior; (5) more hidden emotions such as guilt and self-blame and anxiety about the future; (6) constructive alternatives in the behavioral expression of strong emotions; and (7) concerns regarding attributions, blame, and what will happen in the future. Many of the techniques described above under Counseling Skills may be applied to the group experience. Groups are usually time-limited for 8 to 15 sessions and follow a generalized format.

The following is an example of a general group technique suggested for disaster or crisis groups by the U.S. Department of Health and Human Services (Farberow & Gordon, 1981). The purpose is introduced as a chance for the members to learn about the experiences of the others in divorce, controlling temper, facing natural disaster, etc. The group leader then proceeds to:

1. Ask all the children what happened to them and their families regarding the issue at hand.
2. As the stories appear, ask the children to tell about their own fears (perhaps even act them out in a dramatic play).
3. In the course of the discussion, provide factual information on the disaster (what happened, why).
4. Ask members of the group to take turns being helpers. The children are paired and then take turns, first asking for help with a problem and then acting as helpers with the others' problems.
5. Assign two children as co-leaders to help control restlessness and distractability among the children.
6. Provide the children with paper, plastic materials, clay, or paints and ask them to depict their experiences. Less verbal and younger groups may find these techniques helpful.
7. Various cognitive behavior-modification techniques might be helpful as needed at this point to teach children more constructive self-talk and provide them with interpretations of their situations.

Children are then allowed to talk over the event and their personal reactions to it. More deeply felt emotions with irrational interpretations can then be discussed by the group as well as fears about the future. It is important to remember to disallow any inaccurate accounts of what happened or rumors.

Alternatively, expression of anger or wishes for revenge should be encouraged, and it is often helpful to use drawings or catharsis to facilitate their expression. Relaxation techniques may prove useful if a group is very tense and jumpy.

After a few days to a week, the group's fears should become less intense. At this point discussion regarding how members might behave if a similiar situation came up can be helpful. The leader can then point toward objective sources of concern and discuss what could be done. This activity helps, since many students are preoccupied with fears regarding the incident happening again. If they can feel prepared to face it, these fears may well subside.

When children are very strongly in control of their fears regarding the incident (and this may take months or even years), fears may be openly confronted: visits to the feared location with support for those who had lost most significantly may be helpful.

Parent Groups

Involving parents is uusually a necessary component of crisis intervention. In fact, one of the surest ways to help children is to help the parents resume their functional role after a crisis. Parents need to know what to expect behaviorally from their children and how to manage it. They need to be educated regarding their own personal reactions and how to manage them. At times, telephone contacts are the only avenue to discuss these issues. On other occasions, when a larger group has been affected by crisis, it can be very helpful to bring parents together as a group. Formats can be adapted from those aimed at children, and supportive educational materials can be found in Appendix A of this book.

Anticipatory Guidance

The concept of anticipatory guidance involves preparation or prior training for children who may experience crisis. These interventions fit under primary prevention through education and include the various programs to prevent drug abuse, ward off potential sexual or physical abusers, and provide psychological education and coping education (Mosher & Springthall, 1971; Ivey & Alschuler, 1973; Clay, 1976) for significant stressors such as death education, breakups with girlfriends, etc. This concept was first suggested by Caplan (1964) on the basis of

Lindemann's (1944) research. Many communities have already begun to implement preventive educational programs in the schools as early as the 1950s (Hahn, 1957).

Because the shool is the primary institution, and perhaps the only one, that comes into daily contact with children and parents in the community, it is in a crucial position to provide such programs, especially to children at risk. School personnel, especially teachers, have a thorough understanding of the children, their emotions, and the cultural environment.

What is more, there has been some suggestion in the literature that if teachers and students are not adequately prepared for crisis psychological services during the preimpact period of a crisis, there may be much higher risk (Aharnstam & Woolf, 1975).

Another form of anticipatory guidance is simulation of emergency situations. Such drills have been found to be highly effective in increasing staff attention and motivation and in decreasing anxiety in children during the stressful event (Inbar & Stoll, 1972). This concept is discussed in Chapter 7 of this book in relation to building preparation for a major stressor.

3

Tips and Factual Information for Specific Crises: A Quick Reference

SCHOOL AVOIDANCE AND SCHOOL PHOBIAS

Children and adolescents need to attend school for a number of significant reasons. Probably the most prominent one, however, is that schools are the main vehicle for socialization and interaction with peers. The school serves as a center for structure, social and academic activities, and development of future direction. When a child or adolescent avoids school, it is usually a sign of serious problems.

It is not unusual for children in crisis to attempt to avoid school. One reason for this tendency is fear of leaving the family and separation from the support system. School avoidance may be a symptom of the family's anxiety with the child's leaving the home. Children with an unrealistically high need to achieve may find the academic environment just as capable of provoking anxiety as individuals who are functioning below their peers academically. Following a major disaster or building crisis, many children who were only moderately anxious about school will develop school avoidance patterns.

School staff, of course, must remain flexible when intervening in such problems. However, in the end a firm insistence that children come to school is required. If the pattern directly follows a major disaster or school crisis, anxiety-reducing intervention techniques can be used in counseling sessions. The family often must be given an ultimatum if the pattern continues over an extended period. Allowing the child to stay home may be the path of least resistance in the short run, but with respect to the long-term good of the child, the family, and the community, its consequences can be disasterous.

PHYSICAL AND SEXUAL ABUSE

Incidence

Survey research indicates that between a fourth and a third of the population of the United States has been exposed to one or more unwanted sexual interactions with adults during their childhood (Finkelhor, 1985; Landis, 1956; Russell, 1984 Walters, 1975). Whereas some estimates of sexual abuse of girls have been as high as 38%, it is generally accepted that between 5% and 30% of children have experienced some form of sexual abuse while growing up (Finkelhor, 1985; Landis, 1956; Swift, 1978). Estimates of this type are a continual problem, since sexual abuse goes unreported in the majority of the cases. Some estimates report that up to half of the cases that receive professional attention are not reported to Child Protective Services, even though such reports are required by law.

- Most abusers are well known to the child if not actually family members.
- In most cases that come to the attention of professionals or community agencies, the abuse has been taking place over an extended period of time. This causes a significant therapeutic obstacle in that long-term adjustment problems are frequently in place before the child received any help.
- Despite anything the abuser may promise, without official intervention the abuse will probably continue.
- Currently there is no fairly accurate method to predict which children are at highest risk for abuse, although siblings of sexually abused children appear to have increased risk for abuse. Stepfathers appear to have a greater liklihood for perpetrating abuse (Finkelhor & Hotaling, 1983). Sexual abuse of more than one child is typical in incest cases.
- Neither legal punishment nor counseling alone appears to deter incestuous fathers from continuing sexual abuse.
- Federal and state laws mandate that professionals report sexual abuse or suspected sexual abuse.

Symptoms

Children who are being victimized rarely report the abuse for fear of punishment by the abuser. Instead, other behavior patterns emerge that teachers and other professionals must learn to recognize. Immediate signs include (Burgess & Holmstrom, 1974, 1980; Krasner, Meyer, & Carroll, 1977; Lewis & Sarrel, 1969) phobias, multiple fears, night terrors, regression (e.g., bed-wetting, thumb-sucking), disruption of normal habits, somatic complaints (particularly abdominal pain), preoccupation with sexual matters, and truancy or running away.

Often adults and adolescents continue to be traumatized by the long-standing effects of childhood sexual abuse. Established symptoms include phobias, multiple fears, depression, suicidal behavior, and problems with establishing or maintaining intimate relationships (Herman & Hirschman, 1977; Lewis & Sarrel, 1969; Meiselman, 1978; Steele & Alexander, 1981; Silver, Boon, & Stones, 1983). The more chronic the abuse, the more brutal the abuse, and the closer the perpetrator to the child, the greater the emotional trauma associated with childhood sexual abuse (Burgess & Holmstrom, 1974, 1980; Krasner, Meyer, & Carroll, 1977; Lewis & Sarrel, 1969).

Interventions

Preventative programs have focused primarily on educating all children to identify potentially threatening situations, to understand their rights, and to model and practice methods to handle a sexually intrusive adult. Schools are the primary site for such child training, and many excellent programs have been developed for children.

In the WHO program, methods of intervening with abusers (case monitoring, counseling, removal of the child from the home) have not been systematically evaluated for effectiveness. Monitoring by professionals in the community and at school is widely believed to deter abuse, but it has never been empirically investigated. Counseling approaches include traditional psychotherapies, crisis intervention techniques, and support groups. The ongoing aspect of the self-help groups appears to be a key in the success of some programs (Giarretto, 1981).

Parents United and Daughters and Sons United are both support groups available in many communities that seek to prevent child abuse and support its victims.

Since most cases of sexual abuse come to professional attention only after long-standing victimization has taken place, it is important for those working with children to increase their sensitivity to signs of sexual abuse. Training of professionals involved with children probably needs to be increased so that more victimized children can receive protection and treatment (Swift, 1986). So many cases go unreported that professionals have been accused of being woefully undereducated or of denying symptoms that they see (Finkelhor & Hotaling, 1983). Once abuse comes to the attention of the professional, it is important that it be reported to Child Protective Services, especially if the child verbally expresses that he or she has been abused. In most cases the school-based professional will need to work with legal systems and court-ordered counseling in order best to help the child.

FAMILY VIOLENCE

There is good reason to believe that a number of students in any school will be living in families where physical violence occurs between the parents. Nearly 6 million wives are abused by husbands in any 1 year. The police spend about a third of their time responding to domestic violence calls. Startlingly, wounds resulting from beatings constitute the single major cause of injury to women and the single most common cause of middle-aged women reporting to hospital emergency rooms.

Wife battering, clearly a large problem, is often made more difficult by tendencies within our society to "blame the victim" (Straus, 1981). These women are typically feeling powerless to leave a marriage. When seen for physical or emotional agony, they are told they are behaving hysterically, that they are "crazy," or that they behaved in a manner that provoked a somewhat deserved attack. Even very obvious signs of recurrent abuse are frequently overlooked.

For generations wife beating was considered within the rights of a husband and, although perhaps not the most diplomatic solution to marital disharmony, certainly a private decision made within the confines of each home. Over the course of the past 10 to 20 years, wife beating has moved in the direction of being viewed as an assault just as any other (O'Reilley, 1983).

The typical wife beater in many ways resembles the typical sexual abuser of children: he was abused as a child himself; his condition is worsened by any stressor; he is very emotionally dependent on his wife; he generally denies the problem; he frequently abuses alcohol; and he can be very charming and manipulative, playing off one professional against another once confronted with the problem.

Although presently there is increasing recognition of this problem and increasing support for physically abused wives (Appleton, 1980), only a small number of violent husbands are reported. An isolated mother may well find relationships with adults at her child's school one of the relatively few potential outlets she has available to her. A relationship with a teacher or a school counselor can continue easily for a school year or more and provide the security necessary for a relatively (for this family) intimate relationship.

Most urban communities have a number of women's help facilities that offer services from weekly counseling to legal support to actual residential facilities for transition to independent living or for actual protection from the battering spouse. It is important to put battered individuals and their families directly in touch with these resources and remove yourself from the middle. That is, although you may want to support this situation emotionally, ultimately you are not the one who can offer real services.

Tips to remember for family violence and battering include the following:

- The battered individual will almost always be the wife.
- Her husband, or the batterer, will usually deny the problem or insist that, if there is a problem, it lies with her. He may appear superficially sweet, charming, and well thought of in the community.
- If she confides in you, she will have very mixed feelings about the wisdom of having done so in the future. You may notice that she avoids you or even suddenly "disappears" from day-to-day school functions. Be sure to communicate to her that she can count on your confidentiality. It sometimes helps to mention briefly any friend who had a similar experience and to sympathize with the difficulty of the situation without pitying her.
- The chances are she will take a long period of time to leave her husband or even to pursue community-based help; be patient but set reasonable limits for your own time involvement. Your job lies in encouraging this individual to find the community-based help, not in taking any other responsibility.
- Be prepared for repeating cyclical crises. Frequently the pattern is that help will be sought during the "bad" times and during "better" times the wife will cling to the desperate hope that the violence will not reoccur. Even when it does, she generally does not have faith that she can exist on her own financially or emotionally. It may take years before she makes steps to get therapy or leave the situation.
- You may become very frustrated and angry with the battered party. Resist the temptation to think of her as "hopeless," "crazy" or deserving of such treatment. She is likely terrified, confused, seriously lacking in self-confidence from years of physical and self-esteem battering, completely isolated, and in a great deal of pain.

DEATH AND LOSS*

From ages 3 to 5, the child's concept of death is living under changed circumstances. The sorrow associated with death is essentially that of

*Adapted from Wilson, 1988.

separation. As the child becomes older (ages 6–8), death is seen as some sort of external creature in a concrete sort of cat-and-mouse game: "If you see it coming, you can get away" (Wilson, 1988). Around the age of 9 years, children have attained more of an adult concept of death. The age and concept of death should be taken into acount when one determines how much trauma a child may be experiencing. It is important to remember, however, that even a very young child who may not see death or loss as permanent can be severly traumatized by the separation anxiety.

The research suggests that disruption of the "bonding" process of significant attachment is as traumatic as that from physical wounds (Engel, 1961). Logically, the intensity of the grief reaction seems to be directly related to the closeness of the lost relationship. Children seem to need to go through and successfully resolve the process of mourning accompanying the loss of a significant individual before they are able to redirect their energies toward learning and confronting other developmental tasks (Wilson, 1988). Unresolved loss can certainly take a major toll on relationships even into adulthood, resulting in avoidance of relationships or formation of unstable, tenuous relationships.

The counseling techniques (discussed in Chapter 2) are steps to aid the child in constructively resolving such an interpersonal shock. Other factors relating to adjusting to a death, however, should also be recognized.

The death of a parent is one of the most overwhelming crises that a child can experience. If the basic needs a child has at this time (extra love and support; to remain in a familiar environment with other significant others; solid assurance of safety and continuing care) are not met for vaious pragmatic reasons (a move must be made, the remaining grieving parent is not capable of meeting the extra demands, etc.), the emotional results can be devastating. However, there is some suggestion that if another nurturant adult (offering a similar or superior quality of care to the lost parent) is found and can care for the child, the adjustment is much less traumatic.

Reactions to the death of a parent vary with age (as discussed above). Loss of the parent to the preschooler often results in verbalized, consciously recognized feelings of abandonment. The child may feel guilty about a fantasized role in this death and fear being punished. Elementary-aged children also feel abandoned but tend more toward withdrawal from family and friends. Preadolescents and adolescents openly blame the remaining parent in some fashion and have various somewhat irrational angry reactions at almost everyone in their lives. Internally such a loss results in loss of self-esteem and isolation from peers. Group counseling, especially for adolescents and preadolescents, is often recommended.

Although the loss of a sibling is also a shock to a child, it appears to be mediated to a large extent by the parents' reactions to the sibling death (Brenner, 1984). The surviving child(ren) are often ignored by bereaved parents and supportive relatives. Parents may need to be reminded to find a way to attend to their other children despite the loss. What's more, the death of the sibling should be openly confronted in the family and not swept under the rug. Parents should be encouraged to discuss the death openly and, in most cases, allow the children to view the body at the funeral.

We assume that the loss of a grandparent or friend triggers similar, but less intense, reactions. Such tragic yet less devastating crises can be learning experiences to provide children with a chance to understand death as far as possible and to learn from watching a parent's grieving, and their own possibly mitigated grieving, how to negotiate a loss.

DIVORCE

It is not unusual for children to be in crisis at various points throughout the divorce process. Stressors are perhaps the most severe for children prior to the separation of the parents, as children have been shown to be acutely aware of marital problems (Cantor, 1979; Luepnitz, 1979).

Common patterns include self-blame, feeling different from peers, and heightened sensitivity to interpersonal incompatibility (Kelly & Berg, 1978; Kurdek & Siesky, 1980a, 1980b). Acting out and aggressive behavior frequently become more common (Stolberg, Camplair, Currier, & Wells, 1987); academic performance is often reduced by interfering classroom behavior problems and apparent difficulty with maintaining attention (Guidubaldi, Perry, & Cleminshaw, 1983).

The negative impact of parental separation on children appears to result from changes in the traditional parent–child relationship: caretakers are generally less physically and/or emotionally available to the child, the child experiences stress, and he or she often interprets unavailability as parental rejection resulting in a loss of self-esteem (Stolberg & Anker, 1983). The acquisition of new skills, the negotiation of developmental tasks, and the development of internal controls can be interfered with because of ongoing distress resulting from the divorce experience (Stolberg & Anker, 1983; Wallerstein, 1983; Stolberg et al., 1987). Longitudinal studies indicate that often family situational stress related to divorce peaks 1 year after the initial separation (Hetherington, Cox, & Cox, 1977). The adaptation of the child generally reflects that of the parents. The more stable, available, and emotionally secure the parent, the better the parenting skills and the less trauma for the children. It is not until 2 to 5 years after the divorce that preschool-aged children (at the time of the divorce) generally show marked improvement (Heatherington et al., 1977).

Posttraumatic recovery is true for many children; however, chronic maladjustment is fairly common, especially in boys (Wallerstein & Kelly, 1980). Factors that have been shown to be related to children's stress level and subsequent adjustment to divorce are:

1. The child's perception of divorce (positive or negative), general ability to cope with change, and adaptability of the child to change.
2. A stable social support system (Goldstein, 1981; Heller & Schneider, 1978; Spanier & Castro, 1979).
3. Economic stability.
4. Extent of negatively or positively evaluated environmental change (Stolberg & Anker, 1983; Stolberg et al., 1987).

SUICIDAL THREATS AND ACTIONS

Incidence

The incidence of teen-age suicide has tripled since 1955 and doubled since 1970 according to Vidal (1986). Leder (1987) cited suicide as the second leading cause of death for teen-agers. Several researchers have commented on the percentage of secondary students who have made suicide attempts. A range of 8.4% to 13.0% was found (Harkavy-Friedman, Asnis, Bock, & DiFiore 1987; Smith & Crawford 1986; Ross, 1985). Pfeffer (1986) has predicted a further 94% increase by the year 2000.

Youth suicide has many implications for the schools. School personnel are being called on to assist suicidal students. Legislation has passed in five states addressing the role of the school in prevention. No national legislation has been passed, although a national conference was sponsored by the government in 1985. The question of the responsibility of the schools with regard to youth suicide is not a new one. Stekel, a social scientist, commented to an outbreak of youth suicide in Europe in the early 1900s, "The school is not responsible for the suicide of its pupils, but it also does not prevent these suicides. This is its only, but perhaps its greatest sin" (quoted in Peck, Farberow, & Litman, 1985, p. 158). Few schools are prepared to deal with youth suicide, and very few policies and procedures have been written to clarify the role of school personnel (Harris & Crawford, 1987).

Poland (1989a) outlined a model program for suicide intervention in the schools. Poland pointed out that school personnel have been sued for inadequately supervising suicidal students and being negligent in not obtaining needed psychological or counseling assistance for the student and for not notifying the parents that their child was known to be suicidal. Courts have also found schools without formal prevention programs liable for monetary damages after the suicide of a student. School policies should provide information on the warning signs of suicide so that all school personnel can detect suicidal students and refer them to school personnel who are trained to assess the severity level of a student's symptoms. The most logical personnel to do this are school psychologists or counselors. Preparation needs to be done in advance to work through personal issues and perceived inadequacies in this area and to investigate the various suicidal assessment scales. It may be advisable to rehearse with a colleague or even a drama student.

There is no one scale or set of questions that is recommended for usage with a suicidal student. Davis et al. (1988) reviewed the available instruments and noted the following instruments as the most promising:

1. The Hilson Adolescent Profile developed by Inwald, Brobst, and Morrisey (1987).
2. The Suicidal Ideation Questionnaire developed by Reynolds (1987).
3. The Suicide Probability Scale developed by Cull and Gill (1982).

Hoff (1978) questioned the effectiveness of lethality-assessment scales and instead stressed communication and the establishemnt of rapport with the student.

The following key points are important to remember in working with suicidal students:

- It is understandable to be anxious, but try to remain calm.
- Seek collaboration and support from a colleague.
- Gather case history information from the student.
- Proceed slowly; approach the student as if he or she were planning a trip and ask logical questions.
- Ask specifics about the suicidal plans of the student and the frequency of his or her suicidal thoughts.
- Emphasize that there are alternatives to suicide and that the student is not the first person to feel this way.
- Do not make any deals with the student to keep his or her suicidal behavior a secret.
- Have the student sign a no-suicide contract.

No-Suicide Contracts

No-suicide contracts have been shown to be effective in preventing youth suicide. Our experience has been that out of approximately 5,000 suicidal students who have signed such a contract in the last decade, only two committed suicide. Fourteen other students who did commit suicide were not detected as suicidal by school personnel. The victims did without exception give their friends clues about their suicide plans. Unfortunately, their friends did not get adult help. A no-suicide contract helps the student take control over his or her suicidal impulses and reduces the anxiety of both the student and school psychologist (Mc-Brien, 1983). Contracts should not be used in isolation (Barrett, 1985). Follow-up, monitoring at school, and community services are needed. A sample no-suicide contract appears in Figure 3.1.

Poland (1989a) stressed that major factors in youth suicide are depression, anger, impulsivity, recklessness, drug usage, and gun availability. These stressors are intensifying factors; most youth suicides are precipitated by an event that causes a young person to act on suicidal thoughts. The most common precipitating events are, in order of importance.

1. Arguments with parents.
2. Break-up of a romantic relationship.
3. Loss of a loved one.
4. Extreme humiliation.

School personnel need to be aware of these factors.

I, _____, a student at _____ take
              Name   School

the responsibility for my welfare and agree not to harm myself in any way. I understand that if I am having suicidal thoughs, I agree to call my counselor _____

                                                                     Name

at _____. If I cannot reach him or her, I will call the Crisis
            Phone No.

Hotline at _____, or I will tell an adult and get help for myself.
            Phone No.

_____   _____
     Student   Witness

FIGURE 3.1. An example of a no-suicide contract.

Parent Notification

Parents must be notified at any time that it is believed that a child is suicidal. The question is not whether to call them but, instead, what to say to them. The goal of parent notification is to safeguard the welfare of the student. The school personnel who notifies parents is also protecting him- or herself from liability. School personnel often think that suicidal students will get upset when they find out that their parents are going to be notified. This is not the case, as most students are very relieved that someone is going to help them. It is appropriate to include the suicidal student in the notification conference.

Parental reaction may range from a cooperative response to an attack on the student or the school representative. School personnel should do their best to elicit a supportive reaction from the parents and should discuss the need for increased supervision of the student and the need to remove lethal weapons such as guns. Parents who refuse to acknowledge the seriousness of the suicidal emergency should be encouraged to sign a form indicating that they have been notified and informed of the emergency. If a parent orders the school representative to refrain from interacting with his or her child, it is important that that school representative be up to date on relevant state legislation. Texas, for example, enacted legislation that specifies that parental permission is not required to serve suicidal minors.

Community Services

Parents need to be enfcouraged to seek appropriate community services such as hospitalization or outpatient counseling. School personnel need to refer to private practitioners in the community who are experienced in working with suicidal clients. School personnel cannot assume the responsibility to provide the primary treatment for the student.

Follow-Up

It is essential that school personnel monitor the progress of the student, remind the student of the no-suicide agreement, and communicate the suicidal behavior to others in the school system. If a suicidal student changes campuses, the appropriate counselor or psychologist at the new campus needs to be informed.

4

Crisis Intervention Consultation

CRISIS AND SCHOOL CULTURE

These students, teachers, secretaries, administrators, and counselors are people who frequently work together for many hours each day for many years. When a death, an attack, divorce, or other potentially critical event occurs, it is experienced as if the event occurred in an extended family. Since the incidence of these events has risen so dramatically, it can be expected that students will be asked to cope emotionally again and again with events considered unique and traumatic to the vast majority of the population. It is this personal attachment and involvement that results in excellent schools; and teachers who forewarn us of emotional reactions that can prolong a crisis play an essential role. It is because we care that we develop positive relationships with students and take pride in their achievements and development. It is also this caring that leaves us shocked, overwhelmed, and crushed when crises occurs among those children. Without appropriate training and understanding, a jarring crisis might interfere significantly with our ability to manage effectively. In the long run, lack of training can result in burnout, chronic stress, and depression. Why can this so readily happen?

1. Unrealistic expectations. Crisis by its very definition will always carry with it some surprise and shock. However, most of us working in education expect that crises will not occur with our students or in our schools. A more realistic expectation is that you will encounter at least one crisis every year. Although incidences of crises vary considerably from year to year, we can fairly safely predict which crises the vast

74

majority of classroom teachers and certainly counselors will encounter. These are summarized in chapter 1 of this book.

2. Blaming oneself for the crisis. Guilt-provoking self-talk only saps our energy for managing a crisis. It is important for all crisis staff to refrain from thoughts such as "if only I would have. . . ." Regular reviews of policy and specific cases should systematically provide input for needed change in the system.

3. Lack of education regarding the nature of the particular crisis.

4. Lack of whole school-district planning and coordination resulting in a sense of "operating alone" or having little support from the administration. It is vital to develop policies and procedures in general for crisis intervention but also for particular sorts of crises. Sample policies and procedures are included for each major category of crisis in Appendix A.

5. Lack of communication with and support from the community.

Marcus enrolled in the fourth grade at Martindale school shortly after his family relocated from a neighboring school district. He was placed in a group of classes appropriate to his age and reported grade level, even though the parents did not bring written documentation of his academic progress. The school noted some difficulty with distractability and hyperactivity on the first day. His classroom teacher, Mrs. Stratten, noted that although he appeared academically able and completed most of the classroom work, he somehow seemed "strange," and the other children tended to shy away from him.

Ms. Stratten, Marcus's teacher, was young and energetic. It was the fall semester of her second year as a teacher, and she was glad she had chosen a career in education instead of pursuing more financially rewarding opportunities in her family's business. To Miss Stratten, teaching represented a qualitative improvement over the single-minded focus on financial advancement that her father had advocated over the years. Teaching seemed to her to be a more meaningful task, one that would enable her to help disadvantaged children to grow and that would provide her with a chance to really contribute to society—to make a difference.

Over the course of her first year in education she had learned a great deal. The year was draining, and she had worked long days and into the evening to prepare materials and lessons for her students. Now, beginning her second year, she felt ready to reap some of the benefits of experience.

Since the other children did not offer him much companionship, Marcus hung around the teacher's desk and chatted as much as she would allow. Adult attention was inordinately important to him, and Marcus spent time running errands for his teacher and bringing her little gifts. After a few weeks, Ms. Stratten began to believe that this troubled little boy might just manage in her class after all. Although he was often tearful and "jittery," he was very anxious to please. She concluded that his emotional needs had probably been neglected for years. If she was willing to go out of her way, she reasoned, and give him the attention that he seemed to need so much, surely accelerated academic growth would not be far behind if only Marcus were given the proper support.

Ms. Stratten began to feel herself losing her patience with some of the other faculty. They would alternately laugh at and be irritated by Marcus. She began spending less time in the teacher's lounge. Since she did feel these comments were unprofessional and staff needed to understand more about how to handle Marcus, she began having conferences with the principal regarding how Marcus should be taught.

At the same time Ms. Stratten began to get more and more involved with Marcus's home life. His mother was a single parent struggling to provide for her two children, who seemed to have little time for herself or her children. Miss Stratten began to spend time with Marcus on Saturdays and to spend weekly hours on the telephone advising and consoling his mother. Although this was personally draining, the hope that she was making a real difference in a needy little boy's life motivated her to continue.

One day Marcus came to school and told Ms. Stratten that his mother hit him so hard with a belt that his bottom hurt and he could not sit down. Ms. Stratten called his mother and discussed her very difficult weekend. Marcus's mother was tearful and self-deprecating and Ms. Stratten had to talk with her for a long time to calm her down and support her sense of self-worth and confidence.

This pattern repeated itself with bruises, burns, and one day what appeared to be broken fingers. The P.E. teacher in the building notified the counselor. The counselor called child welfare. When the investigation began it became clear that this was not the first time such a report had been made.

At that point, everything fell apart for Miss Stratten. The principal and the child protection staff after questioning became aware that previous incidents had not been reported by her. Both were critical of her behavior, which was considered in violation of the law. She received a negative evaluation and was put on professional probation for the subsequent academic year. The faculty already alienated by Ms. Stratten's directions concerning Marcus's treatment, showed little support. In fact, Ms. Stratten felt that she noticed that conversations ended abruptly whenever she entered the teacher's lounge. Marcus's mother became angry and accusatory with Ms. Stratten for "meddling in their family life" and "not sticking to her job as a teacher." Even Marcus told her she was a "bad lady" because she got his mother in trouble, and that he did not want to see her anymore.

Miss Stratten questioned her choice of career and a system that would persecute someone for trying so hard to help a child, and spent many tearful nights. The following year she left the teaching profession.

BASIC CONSULTATION SKILLS

Consultation skills are an essential key in this second approach, and they are distinct from general clinical or counseling skills. Many psychologists with excellent skills in individual, family, and group therapy find they are running up against a brick wall when faced with intervention in a system such as a school district. For this reason some of the basic elements of the consultative role are outlined below.

Table 4.1 summarizes some of the more significant aspects of the consultative style (reproduced from Conoley & Conoley, 1982). There are several clear differences from the "psychologist as expert" or "doctor" posture of many clinical approaches.

Whether the school psychologist operates out of a private office or is a full-time district employee, whether he or she functions in a more traditional role of special-education-bound testing or operates more

TABLE 4.1. Aspects of the Consultative Style

1. Consultee initiated
2. Consultee has complete freedom to accept or reject services (the relationship can be terminated by consultee at any point)
3. Confidentiality of relationship
4. Peer–professional collaborative relationship (consultant viewed as facilitative role, not expert role)
5. Indirect resource service
   a. Economy of service
   b. Generalizability of service
   c. Long-term effects
6. Work-related problems only
7. Primary prevention orientation (acute and chronic problems are dealt with as well)
8. Goals of the consultant
   a. Provide an objective point of view
   b. Help to increase problem-solving skills
   c. Help to increase coping skills
   d. Help to increase freedom of choice
   e. Help to increase commitment to choices made
   f. Increase resources available on persistent problems.

Source: Conoley & Conoley (1982).

flexibly, the consultation model is probably going to be a key if crisis intervention (tertiary prevention) or prevention (primary and secondary prevention) is to be promoted in the school district. If your approach is that of an expert who will teach the district "how to do it right," the chances are high that a continuing, collaborative relationship will not occur. If, after having received an initial invitation for involvement, you approach district personnel as "let's put our heads together to see if we can avoid some of these problems next time" or "some other districts have had some nice ideas to avoid this sort of thing; want to see what you think?" it may be the beginning of a long and constructive collaboration.

Many psychologists working in the schools are concerned regarding limits on their role. The activities reported most commonly that limit their functioning include attending meetings, testing, and being tied to special education funding.

Criteria for Use of Crisis Case Consultation*

1. A particular school employee may wish to provide a service for a person in crisis in which he or she is not particularly skilled.
2. An administration experienced in managing crises wants to obtain a broader, more preventive perspective and establish an organized system for crisis management.
3. Administration needs a crisis counselor to intervene in staff crises.
4. Specific educational functions possibly relating to training in suicide prevention, running divorce groups, etc.
5. Individuals in need of the support of a colleague.

Program Consultation

"Case" consultation is probably the most common consultative sort of referral. This type of consultation involves working with groups of individuals regarding a certain topic (e.g., assessing suicidal clients) or an individual student. "Program" consultation is presently practiced much less frequently (Anderson, 1976). Often it is only after a crisis occurs that administrators and staff feel it necessary to review the program and institutions that contribute to crisis.

CONSULTATION REGARDING THE CONTROL OF OTHERS
Avoiding a Conflict Cycle

Control of students and even other adults in the schools is an integral part of the school classroom. Teachers are expected to control their

*Adapted from Hoff (1978).

classrooms. Principals are expected to keep control of their student bodies and of their teaching staff. If a rowdy, difficult-to-manage student is present, he must be kept under control. Somehow and somewhere in the dim childhood memories of most us lies a basic reflexive, almost instinctive reaction to challenges to our authority or self-confidence. For many of us, a great deal of emphasis is placed on being in control and a sense of being able to control others. We begin to have a sense of taking control of our lives, keeping control of our children, not letting our mate "get away" with anything. Likewise, we lead ourselves to believe that if we are to be successful in the workplace we must control those around us. We must control our employees, we must control our clients, and, perhaps most emphatically, to be successful, we must control the children we work with.

How this control is to be achieved is often a "knee-jerk" automatic reaction. Often it involves applying skills we have learned from our parents prior to conscious speech, a reaction that is partly emotional, partly instinctual, and largely not well thought out in advance. Nowhere in our experience do these basics of psychology get played out so dramatically as in the school. Very often administrators and teachers make statements like:

"I won't have that!"
"You can't pull that on me!"
"My child, husband, friend wouldn't get away with that!"

These statements all suggest that somehow one can control others to disallow or remove a particular behavioral pattern. The behavioral manifestation of this process most often translates into aggressive, threatening tactics. What if someone doesn't behave as you expect or demand? You might first issue a firm order: "Don't do it." The second attempt might be coupled with an order and a threat: "Don't do it or you'll be sorry." Further escalation might include raising your voice, refusing to cooperate with requests made by the individual (a form of extortion), refusal to speak to the individual (the traditional "silent treatment"), or angry or tearful emotional outbursts often combined with personal attacks (the traditional "telling someone off"). All of these behavioral patterns are manipulative attempts to "force" someone to behave as you wish. All of these behavioral patterns are attempts to "control" the individual.

What we often fail to recognize is that even if the individual complies with our demands, we did not "make" him or her do anything. With a little pressure that person has decided to give in—and probably not without resentment.

If we have had a good deal of success with these techniques in the classroom and in our personal lives, we probably execute the pattern without even being fully conscious of our goals and manipulative tactics. It is possible that escalation and threat have met our needs in controlling individuals for many years. In schools these techniques for managing children and adolescents are used frequently by individuals in authority. In the past if the child or adolescent did not respond to them, he or she was labeled "no good" or "hopeless" and kicked out.

Children and adolescents with behavioral and emotional problems often do not respond to these intimidating techniques. If we do not recognize totally that the individual we are attempting to control has in the past *chosen* to comply but instead attribute our successes to sheer power or control on our own part, we have the potential to greatly escalate any conflict. If one believes that power and intimidation control inappropriate behavior and encounters someone for whom this is not true (someone who choses not to comply when these techniques are used and who might respond with incredibly higher levels of intimidating behavior), the situation begins to evolve quickly into a crisis with escalating, out-of-control behavior on both sides.

In a situation involving adult peers, such escalations are characterized by angry verbal exchanges; people make statements that they don't mean and later regret. Marital couples find themselves furious and tearful. Each is attempting to effect a behavioral change in the other, using the methods that worked so well in childhood or in their own nuclear families. Both see it as necessary to continue to escalate and threaten, "up the ante", if you will, and both are in sufficient emotional crisis that the relationship, the feelings of the loved one, and their long-term goals are sacrificed in an attempt to "win," to "dominate." Parents who sacrifice their relationship with their adolescent children because their bedrooms are not orderly fall into this same category as do some teachers with their students.

These cycles are acted out in the schools more often than any other institution. Adults are attempting to control children. Many children with behavioral problems, self-control problems, emotional problems, etc., escalate in the face of intimidation. If the psychologist and the staff cannot use alternative control means to short-circuit this process, many "scenes" will occur that might have been prevented.

Managing Verbal and Physical Aggression

It is not the place of the psychologist or the administrative staff to take primary responsibility for physically apprehending an individual. If a crime is being committed, the police are the appropriate interveners. If the school district involved has security (which roughly half now report having on staff), they are the more appropriate interveners.

With this point made quite emphatically, it is also true that any psychologist or other school staff members who works with crisis intervention or at-risk populations eventually will be confronted with physical violence, perhaps involving a weapon. Anyone who does attempt to overpower a student or intruder should do so only with appropriate training. This training is equally essential for staff working with "high-risk" groups of students such as the emotionally and behaviorally disturbed, mentally handicapped, neurologically damaged, attention deficit, hyperactive-disordered individuals, autistic pervasive developmental-disordered individuals, and alternative-program students who may have been removed from the regular placement because of substance abuse, verbal and physical violence, or other juvenile crimes. This is equally true for young children as it is for adults.

It is indispensable for these psychologists to have a clear understanding of how physically to protect themselves, to avoid placing themselves in situations in which uncontrollable physical aggression might occur, and, when absolutely necessary, how physically to manage an out-of-control person. It is beyond the scope of this book to describe the motions and holds involved in physically protecting oneself or overpowering another person. What's more, these skills are best learned in an "in vivo" setting with modeling and practice as essential components of the learning process. There are, however, some general guidelines involving physically aggressive behavior that can be addressed.

Many local and national groups are springing up that specialize in training a variety of professionals (police, psychologists, teachers, juvenile workers, security officers, and mental health workers) in the area of managing verbal and physical aggression. One of these, the National Crisis Prevention Institute, conducts annual workshops on identifying, preventing, and managing physically and verbally aggressive behavior across the nation.

Perhaps the most complicated judgment to make is the determination of when physical intervention is not necessary and when it is immediately necessary. As the crisis unfolds, the anxiety of everyone involved begins to escalate. As this occurs, the physiological "fight or flight" reaction is triggered: hearts race, faces become flushed, muscles tense, breathing quickens. It can be a challenge to make logical, carefully thought out decisions in this state, but if one has prior training, it can also be an advantage, as shown in Table 4.2 (National Crisis Prevention Institute Conference, 1986).

Individuals who are likely to face crises must be taught to control their anxiety in order to maximize the advantages of fear and anxiety. With

TABLE 4.2. Reactions to Fear and Anxiety

Nonproductive	Productive
Freezing	Increased speed and strength
Over-underreacting (either motorically or rationally)	Increased sensory acuity
	Decreased reaction time
Inappropriately aggressive reaction physically (attacking, punching) or verbally (unprofessional language, name calling)	

support, training, and experience, individuals begin to increase their self-confidence in managing the potential confrontations involved in crises. This "know-how" then serves to minimize the stress and burnout associated with chronic crisis-oriented positions.

Probably the mainstay of controlling anxiety is the secure knowledge that you (and those working with you) can completely overpower the potentially physically violent individual if necessary. This should be obvious to the individual who is acting out also. Never enter into or even imply that you would enter into physical confrontation unless there is no question that the necessary strength to quickly physically overpower the acting-out individual is present. If it is not obvious to all involved, steps must be taken to correct the situation. More security might be called, or often a few extra adults standing in the vicinity will quickly communicate to the potentially violent individual that he or she can quickly be overpowered. Often this is enough to produce compliance.

Individuals who work in an ongoing capacity with students or adults prone to crisis do themselves a great favor by removing potential weapons from the environment. Necklaces, scarves worn around the neck and head, hoop earrings, rings, and long fingernails should be eliminated from the work wardrobe. Long hair should be up and fastened tightly to the head. Clip-on ties are strongly recommended for men.

Much of the time it is possible to avoid the use of physical overpowering. Frequently a series of verbal escalations occurs before the actual physical acting out. Different management techniques are associated with each of the stages of escalation (see Table 4.3). An individual attempting to manage a crisis must have the skills to discriminate among these subtleties of behavior and modulate his or her own reaction in accord if the situation is to be managed effectively.

Frequently generalized anxiety is the forerunner of behavioral escalation. If you have been working with crisis-prone individuals for any

TABLE 4.3. Stages in Escalation to Physical Aggression

Symptom or behavior	Management reaction
Anxiety	Supportive: active listening
Mildly verbally aggressive or defensive	
Loss of logical thinking	Do not expect logic or point out the illogical aspects
Questioning of authority	Determine whether question is legitimate; don't answer those that are not
Refusal to cooperate, comply with authority's requests	State two or three choices and the associated consequences
Severely verbally aggressive verbal "dumping"	Wait until the individual wears him- or herself out; do not change the limits or rules you have set up
Irrational, out-of-control release	
Attempts at intimidation	Take threats seriously; avoid showing fear
Physical acting out	Therapeutic holding; removal

Note: Adapted from National Crisis Prevention Institute (1986).

length of time, you will recognize such familiar comments as "I can tell what kind of day we are going to have by his mood when he walks in the door" or "If he's disappointed in something, the rest of the day is nothing but a conflict." Experienced faculty can often see trouble coming by signs of anxiety. If there is an appropriate time for a supportive approach, individual attention, active listening, and leniency, it is now. The student at this point is concerned, worried, frightened, or overwrought. This is an appropriate point to consider measures to reduce the tension such as time alone, taking a break, getting a hug (for young children), a smile, or a pat on the back. Hopefully, through these methods, the skilled staff members can derail any potential escalation.

The inexperienced individual may react to anxiety-based behavior in the child with increased anxiety of his or her own, especially if escalation has occurred in the past. If the crisis manager is not careful, his or her very behavior can escalate that of the student. His or her voice may rise in volume, become staccato, or adopt an adversarial tone. He or she may take a hands-on-hips, squared-off challenging posture. The student's space may be invaded. Any approach that is likely to escalate the anxiety of the student is likely to escalate the levels of verbal and physical violence, especially if the student is prone to acting out as a coping mechanism.

The supportive posture, however, must quickly change once the first signs of aggression occur. By answering inappropriate, challenging questions, the crisis manager allows the escalating individual to gain confidence and to gain a sense of controlling the situation. This sense of control frequently leads to increased acting out. A brief answer to legitimate questions (often it is no simple task to make this discrimination) is necessasry. Questions such as the following deserve a brief response:

> Where am I supposed to be now?
> It's lunchtime, right?
> What am I supposed to be working on?
> Where is Toni?
> Where is my mother?
> Can I go to the office?

Alternatively, questions or provocative statements such as the following do not deserve a response or discussion:

> What kind of teacher are you, anyway?
> Can you explain what the hell you are doing?
> Don't you know what you are doing?
> You don't care about us—you're just here for a paycheck.
> You can't tell me what to do.
> I'll do what I damn well place, asshole.
> My mother is going to sue all of you.

A simple directive should be repeated at reasonable intervals in a calm, natural voice to the above responses. It is helpful for the intervener to redirect his or her attention to another nearby task while giving verbal directives and consequences. This accomplishes a number of objectives: (a) it allows personal space for the escalating individual; (2) it allows a "safety" space for the intervener without sending out the message that he or she is "afraid" or "on the run"; and (3) it permits the (often) reinforcing attention to be withdrawn momentarily. If the crisis individual deescalates at this point, it may be constructive to reward the choice with closer proximity and eye contact if this is not disturbing to the individual.

Behavioral choices and consequences for the choices often require some thought in advance. Both the choices and the consequences must be concrete and *enforceable*. Emotional statements such as "get to work or I'll have your hide" may be appropriate in a less emotionally charged situation, but they sound like little more than hollow threats during a crisis. Likewise, "if you break that, you won't ever set foot in this building again" often has the effect of a challenge, daring the individual to try the forbidden activity. Statements such as "if you decide to break it, you will stay after school and work until it is paid for" generally carry a more sobering effect.

Alternatively, the individual in crisis may, at this point, escalate to complete loss of verbal control, which usually includes a long, irrational tirade. Attempts to "shut him or her up" or break into the speech usually result in further escalation—the crisis individual either runs from the premises or, more typically, engages in some sort of physical acting out. The tirade should not be interupted. It is important to let the individual in crisis "burn him- or herself out." When this occurs, it is hoped that much of his or her anger, anxiety, and pent-up emotion will be gone with it.

It is not unusual for such a tirade to be triggered by the threat of undesired consequences or choices from the previous stage. If this is the case, the managing individual may feel pressure to give in and grant a different, more acceptable alternative, especially if undesirable threats are involved. Under no circumstances should this be done. Although it is possible that the individual in crisis may calm down when the pressure is reduced, he also gets the message that with a few intimidation tactics, he is in control. The more control the individual feels, the greater the probability that in the future, or even in the present situation, he or she will consider you a safe target for acting out.

Threats made by the individual in crisis should be acknowledged and taken seriously. Such statements as "I could just bash your face in" and "Don't forget, I know where you live" should not be responded to with laughter, minimizing comments, or even a casual brush-off. Usually the threatening individual carefully watches the intervener for traces of fear, shock, etc. Such threats must be anticipated by those who will be managing crises, who must contain personal emotional reactions as much as possible. However, steps should definitely be taken to protect oneself, such as isolating the crisis individual or calling in additional staff or security as necessary.

Much of the intervention in the face of threatened physical aggression runs contrary to a therapeutic environment, where ventilation is often encouraged. In a crisis situation, the intervener must function as an authority figure. The intervener is not solely authoritarian but reinforces by expression, tone, and gesture behaviors on the part of the acting-out individual that will serve to resolve the crisis. The student is given choices by the crisis manager and team to encourage him or her to take responsibility for his or her own actions.

Those psychologists with training and experience limited to more traditional therapeutic venues will need to cultivate a distinctly different set of skills in this area of crisis intervention. This more authoritarian role may not be what most of us imagined when we chose a career in psychology; neither did most administrators, teachers, or counselors. These skills, however, are becoming quite indispensable when one is working in the schools, and it does no one any favors to deny their necessity, much as victims of crisis themselves are prone to deny what is happening.

Intervention in a Fight

For years school personnel have been faced with the question of how much they should get involved to break up a fight. Many staff members have been injured while attempting to break up a fight. A Montana teacher at in-service described how a teacher had jumped between two students who were fighting. The teacher was cut with a knife and exchanged blood with the two students. Although not injured seriously, the teacher did demand that both students submit to testing for the AIDS virus. The students refused.

Students who are fighting or brandishing weapons in the schools cause an emotional reaction in all of us (Fischer & Sorenson, 1985). As the Supreme Court Justice Oliver Wendell Holmes succinctly stated, "Detached reflection cannot be expected in front of an uplifted knife." Faced with such an extreme threat to physical safety, school personnel cannot be expected to provide the same forethought and care as during a nonviolent confrontation.

A large 17-year-old student, drunk and agitated, arrived at the separate campus for behavior-problem students. The program director told him that he could not be in school; he was to wait outside for his mother, who would be called. The student refused and crashed through a classroom window to reenter school. He suffered cuts to his arms. The teacher calmly told the student to follow him into the hall. All teachers heard the commotion, locked their doors, and told students to stay in the classroom and away from the high windows, although the other students were eager to get involved. The agitated and injured student was isolated in the hallway with the teacher. The program director and I went out to help. I thought, "I am a psychologist; I should be able to help." I approached the student and said what I thought were calming words. The student interpreted them differently and swung at me. I stepped back and stopped talking. The teacher began talking to the student in a very calm and almost inaudible voice. The student strained to hear what was being said. The student noticeably calmed down and eventually even asked to be allowed to wait in the time-out place until his mother arrived. The incident would have been calmly resolved had not another student agitated the belligerent student and the police who then arrived at the school. Unfortunately, the result was that both students resisted arrest and had to be physically subdued and handcuffed. The police could have deescalated the situation with a different approach, especially if they had used the involved teacher to help calm the students.

This example illustrates two key points about intervening with violent individuals: (1) remove the audience; and (2) whoever knows the violent individual best should intervene. Usually, then, it is not the school psychologist who is the individual of choice to intervene. A consultative role is, in most cases, the most productive for school psychology.

Of course, prevention is the first-choice solution. The previous two chapters of this book relate to prevention of violence in the general sense. However, if a fight is imminent, the intervener can first attempt to offer other ways to cope with the angry, violent emotions. It may be helpful to watch for physiological clues to determine when a violent individual is about to act (Moss, 1989). These include palpitations at the temple and carotid arteries, constriction of the pupils, clenching of the jaw muscles, flaring of the nostrils, and indentation of the muscle groups in the neck and chest.

Other recommendations that are helpful to school personnel (Leviton & Greenstone, 1989; Martin, 1989) include step-by-step guidance, as follows:

- *Don't rush* to the scene. Hurrying to the scene appears warranted only if it offers the opportunity of intervening before the fight starts (Glenn, 1990). If it is possible to delay a fight, try. Violence has a time line, and *the longer the violence is delayed, the less chance it will occur* at all. If the fight is already in progress, walk to the scene and observe closely before taking action.
- *Get help and prepare* along the way. It may be smart to remove jewelry, other sharp objects, or potentially dangerous possessions (e.g., long scarves or dangling clothing).
- When you arrive at the scene, *analyze* the situation. Remove obstacles or potential weapons around the violent individuals, locate the exit, and avoid being cornered.
- *Announce your presence.* Avoid physical attempts to stop the fight. Move slowly, initiate eye contact with the violent individuals, and monitor their facial rections. Maintain a distance of at least 2 or 3 feet, have hands ready to deflect blows, and avoid turning your back to the violent individuals.

- *Call the students by name.* Use your voice as a tool. It is important to remember that the violent individuals are angry, so the intervener must stay calm, caring, and empathetic (Leviton & Greenstone, 1989).
- *Give the clear, simple order to stop fighting.*
- *Try humor* to distract the students (e.g., "Bill, what did you have for lunch—the chili's giving everybody gas!").
- *Don't threaten* the violent individuals with consequences; instead give them choices (e.g., "You may go see the nurse or the counselor; you may not stay here and fight"). Be aware of your nonverbal posture (as above).
- *Don't be a hero*—school personnel need not feel it is their job to break up fights.
- *Document* the fight and contact parents and possibly police or juvenile authorities as soon as possible.

CONSULTATION INVOLVING A DEATH AT SCHOOL

Statistics suggest (Stevenson, 1986) that one of every 750 school children dies each year. This sadly means that all educators will be dealing with the death of a student at some point. Administrators may want to ignore the impact of the death or to rush too quickly to return to normality.

Students and teachers need to process the death, and having possessions of the deceased helps them to do so. We have observed schools rushing to remove the personal possessions, artwork, desks, etc., of deceased students. Teachers sometimes feel that rearranging desks will help students when a classmate dies. This only adds to the emotional turmoil.

One particularly striking example took place after the murder of a grade-school student (Poland & Pitcher, 1989). The principal came to school early and removed all of the deceased student's possessions including her desk. He instructed the teacher not to allow the students to talk about this classmate's death. The teacher and fellow classmates were angered and confused by the actions of the principal. One stated, "I know we are not supposed to talk about her death, but couldn't we at least go out on the playground and let balloons go in her memory?" The teacher accepted this, and the class did so. The teacher later noted that the ceremony helped the students let go of their deceased classmate and represented for most of them her spirit ascending to heaven.

No matter how heinous the incident, it is much more productive and realistic to face the situation from the onset. An incident in New York

(Lipton, 1990) involved a principal's refusal to deal with murder in front of the school. Students at an elementary school saw a body in front of the school and homicide detectives investigating the crime scene. The students wanted to know what had happened. When students went to the principal and asked what had happened, the principal denied that there had been a murder and told the students to look out of the window. The sidewalk was vacant; the body had been removed. The principal said, "See, nothing happened in front of our school; now go on back to class." The students were confused and angrily returned to the principal's office the next day armed with the newspaper article describing the murder in front of their school. The principal then had no choice but to acknowledge the murder.

School-Wide Reactions

Reactions of the school as a whole seem to vary significantly in response to death. School employees often report that they had underestimated the degree of trauma when the death of a popular faculty member or student occurred. Other schools have been surprised by the minimal impact that the death of a new student had on the student body as a whole.

Consider the following examples:

- A 16-year-old boy hung himself at home less than 1 mile from the high school. He had recently moved to the area and never enrolled at school. His death had little impact on the school.
- A 15-year-old boy shot himself in math class in front of 24 students. He was not a popular, well-known student, but because the death had occurred at school, it was very traumatic for the entire school community.
- A very well-liked principal who had been with the district for many years died of cancer only days after the school had heard he was getting better. His death was very traumatic.
- The third employee at an elementary school died of natural causes within the same school year. Two of the employees were fifth-grade teachers. The students had liked all the employees but had especially worshipped the third teacher who died, and many felt that he had been the best teacher that they had ever had. The third death was very traumatic and brought up lots of unresolved issues from the first two deaths.

Three key questions are helpful in estimating the severity of the school reaction when a death occurs (Oates, 1988):

1. *Who* was the person? How popular and well known was he or she? Has the person been in the community or on the campus for a long time?
2. *How* did the individual die? Murder and suicide are more violent, unexpected, and sudden and will create more trauma than a natural death will.
3. *Where* did the death occur? A death that occurs at the school will be more traumatic to deal with.

A fourth question that we recommend asking is:

4. What other deaths have occurred in your school community recently?

These questions have proven very useful in determining the degree of trauma and deciding how much intervention (counselors, psychologists, etc.) might be needed following a death.

Actions to Take Following a Death

The death must be acknowledged and rumors dispelled. Students and teachers need to talk about the death. Teachers need to model expression of emotion and allow students a range of emotions. Tips for teachers after a death in any crisis are outlined in Appendix A. The following questions will need to be answered:

1. Should a faculty meeting be held? Yes, as soon as possible. A calling tree could alert people the night before and announce a staff meeting before school. School personnel have commented that it helps them to get the news the night before. This allows them to prepare for the next school day.
2. How should the death be announced? Our preference is for a memorandum written by the principal and hand delivered to teachers providing specific facts about what has happened and instructions regarding how they should interact with the students.
3. What about public address announcements of a death? This can be acceptable in some circumstances. The announcement should be carefully worded and rehearsed by the person reading it. The announcement should also encourage teachers to keep the majority of students (prefereably 98%) in their classroom. One principal announced that any student who wished more details about the death should come to the auditorium. It was estimated that over 200 students came, and it proved difficult to manage such a large group.
4. What about the classes that the deceased would have attended? Someone should follow the schedule of the deceased to answer questions

that his or her classmates might have and to allow for expression of emotions.

5. What activities should be provided for students to help them ex-1press emotions? Classroom discussions, small-group counseling, individual counseling, written expression, art and music activities, and cards, letters, and projects to assist the family are all appropriate activities to foster such expression. Sample activities are provided in Appendix A.

6. Are there certain books that could be read to children following a loss? Yes. A list of recommended books appears in Appendix F.

7. How much contact should there be with the parents of the deceased? The school should reach out and assist the family for a number of reasons. One of these is that there almost always are surviving children who attend your schools.

8. Should the school contact the families of students who are upset? Yes, one of the ways that we help students the most is through assisting their parents.

9. Does it help students to make a list of positive things about the deceased? Yes, students should be encouraged to share positive memories of the deceased.

10. Are there certain "magic" words that should be said to students? No. Acknowledge the death, express emotions and thoughts, and then get the students to talk. It is very important to be sincere, warm, and empathetic. Students have commented to us when the group leader appeared cold and uncaring. If the group leader did not know the student, it should be acknowledged through a statment such as, "I didn't know Bill. But I'd like to know about him. Please tell me about him."

11. Should the curriculum be set aside in certain classes? Yes, the administrator should clearly give permission to set aside academics, and the return to them should be gradual.

12. Should school be dismissed because of the death of someone? No, students will get the most help with their emotions at school with their classmates, teachers, counselors, etc. School should be held with creative use of time and facilities. Scheduled extracurricular activities should be held.

13. What about funeral attendance? Students who wish to attend the funeral should be allowed to do so. Their parents should be encouraged to accompany them. Students also need to ask questions about the funeral and should anticipate and prepare for it. Many students have never attended a funeral. Students may also need to process the funeral experience when they return to school.

14. Should school be dismissed for the funeral? This is a difficult question to answer. It depends on the circumstances—who the person was, and what happened? If it was a suicide, then school should *not* be dismissed (Poland, 1989a).

15. What if a student has a severe reaction to the death? The parents

of the student need to be notified and encouraged to seek community assistance such as private counseling for their child.

16. Do students at different ages react differently to a death? Yes, children go through definite developmental stages as they learn the meaning of death. These stages are discussed in greater detail in Poland (1989a).

17. What size should a counseling group be to help students deal with the death? Five to eight is ideal, but it may be necessary to work with up to 20 students. Space needs to be located so that students can be assisted in small groups.

18. Will some students take advantage of the tragedy? Yes, and we need to set limits for them, but it is better to have a few students take advantage than to forbid anyone to express his or her emotions. After several hours all students need to be encouraged to return to class. Stress that it is permissible to cry in class and that there may be another person whom they can assist.

19. Should schools bring in outside assistance such as private counselors and local clergy? This decision should be made prior to a death or any crisis. The professionals who are going to provide outside assistance should be formally interviewed individually and then placed on a team. The outside assistance team should then meet and coordinate plans to invervene in a crisis. Consideration needs to be given to the availability of school personnel such as counselors and psychologists. In general it is recommended that school personnel handle the death. There can be complicated issues involved when private practitioners and clergy come to school, due to competition and differences in philosophy.

CONSULTATION REGARDING SCHOOL SAFETY
Legal Issues

Several areas that deal with how schools interface with public agencies, such as police and courts, have been questioned recently. At least one state, California, has addressed constitutionally a student's right to attend safe schools. In addition, the liability of the school district or administration with regard to violence and youth suicide has been extended in recent court decisions.

Right to Safe Schools

California passed a constitutional amendment in 1982 stating that all students have an inalienable right to attend campuses that are safe, secure, and peaceful. Sawyer (1985) emphasized that the amendment outlined that students have a right to be protected from the following:

- Crime, violence, and criminal activity.
- Identifiable dangerous students.
- Negligently admitted or placed dangerous students.
- Negligently selected trained administrators or teachers.

The amendment also called for harsher penalties for those who commit crimes at school. In addition, the amendment raised the possibility that if the local school board could not make the schools safe, the courts might step in and take control. This apparently never has taken place but might be similar to the state appointing a master to run a school system after academic accreditation has been revoked. It is difficult to know exactly what such legislation actually means for a student in California. Sawyer stressed the common-sense approach that the amendment emphasized and cautioned schools that lack of funds is not a sufficient reason for not taking steps to make schools safer. Turner (1989) discussed a court ruling that upheld the principle of safe schools but did not specify rules or an express duty of anyone to make them safe. It is a promising but complicated area for state legislatures to address. At this writing, we are aware of some similar legislation in other states. For example, South Carolina has passed legislation requiring each school to have a crisis plan.

Coordination Between the Schools and the Judicial System

School districts have historically operated independently of the judicial system. Principals sometimes say, "Son, what you have done is so serious that you are being expelled from school, but I am going to do you a favor and not report your crime to the police." This sets up a double standard for the student. That same administrator may express frustration that the judicial system does not take action when the young offender is reported at a later date. The judicial representative might then say, "You mean he has brought a gun to school three times before. I am sorry that you didn't report the other three incidents. Since I have no official record of them, I will not be able to take judicial action." Goldsmith (1988) commented, "Until juvenile records are uniformly shared among professional educators, law enforcers, and social workers, youths will continue to beat and get beat by the system" (p. 18). Goldsmith described a data-base-sharing system utilized in Indianapolis. Clontz (1988) addressed the question of how schools can gain access to the juvenile justice records of the students. Schools have been added to the list of those that do not need a court order to get a copy of the juvenile justice records in some states. The NSSC has copies of model state legislation to coordinate efforts between the school and the judicial system. Statistics should be kept concerning crime and violence at school. Certainly, everyone can plan better to alleviate problems if it is known exactly what course they have taken in the past and their current status.

We have been frustrated in our own district when we have tried to facilitate working with probation and parole officers. Often we cannot find out who is on probation or parole and if we do find out which students are, then either we cannot identify the assigned judicial representative or cannot get him or her to work with us. The judicial system tells the student to go to school and do a good job but never checks up on its charge. The following scenario is typical:

> Bob had been placed on a lengthy and supposedly strict probation. His school attendance and behavior were unacceptable. Bob repeatedly threatened to harm his teachers. The principal, after much effort, located the probation officer. The probation officer not only thought that Bob had been doing well in school but also thought that he attended a regular high school. Bob in fact had been placed on a separate campus in an alternative program years before. The probation officer came to school and met with Bob and school personnel and told Bob to straighten up or he was going to jail. Bob's school performance improved immediately.

Why Don't Administrators Report Crime?

"Historically, our nation's schools have distanced themselves from the criminal justice system" (Staff, 1988, p. 107). The most commonly cited explanations by administrators for unreported crimes, according to Rapp, Carrington, and Nicholson (1986), were the following:

- Wish to avoid publicity and litigation.
- Fear they will be viewed as ineffective.
- Perception of some offenses as too minor to report.
- Preference for relying on their own discipline system.
- Suspicion the police and courts would not cooperate.

The reasons that teachers do not report crime were similar:

- Fear of being blamed or retaliation from the student.
- Desire to avoid litigation.
- Trouble identifying the offender.
- Desire not to stigmatize the young offender.

Rapp et al. (1989) emphasized that school boards, although outraged at student crime and violence, did not feel responsible for eliminating the problem.

Legal Trend to Hold Third-Party Defendents (Schools) Liable

Turner (1989) discussed *Hosemann versus the Oakland, California schools.* School officials were aware that a student had repeatedly bullied Hosemann but took no action to warn Hosemann. Hosemann was injured by the student, and his parents filed suit. The first court found the school liable and awarded monetary damages and ordered the school to develop a crisis plan. The Oakland schools appealed the decision, and the Appeals Court overturned the ruling, citing that no rules exist as to how schools are to be made safe.

Similar cases involving liability specific to youth suicide have occurred. Slenkovitch (1986) discussed *Kelson versus Springfield, Oregon schools.* Kelson, who had robbed his teacher, was known to be suicidal and to have a gun in his possession. Kelson had pleaded with the assistant principal and the police to speak with the school counselor. His request was refused. Kelson was allowed to go to the restroom unsupervised, where he shot himself to death. His parents filed a lawsuit, and the school district settled out of court for a large amount of money. Poland (1989a) addressed the key questions in this and other similar cases:

1. Should school officials have been able to *foresee* that Kelson was at risk?
2. Were reasonable steps taken to prevent the suicide?
3. Is it negligent not to get psychological help for a suicidal student?

A court in Munster, Indiana awarded $50,000 in damages to the parents of a boy who committed suicide. The court said that the school was negligent in not notifying the parents that their son had threatened suicide (Suicide ruling not be be appealed, 1989). The Kelson case and the one from Munster, Indiana emphasize the need for schools to have suicide-prevention policies in place and the need to train school personnel to detect and assist suicidal students.

Should Schools Have Their Own Police or Security Personnel?

Suburban and urban schools frequently have campus or district security personnel. Some of these personnel are commissioned as police officers and can make arrests. Others are not commissioned as police officers. Some commissioned officers wear uniforms and carry guns. Our own district has debated the need for school police. A common school response to frequent violence is to hire additional security personnel. Is that the answer and the best use of funds? Are schools reluctant to hire their own police force and face the reality of violence at school? These are difficult questions to answer and need to be debated by the school board or an administrative committee. One obvious benefit in having a school police force is that it can coordinate with local law enforcement, as outlined in Appendix A.

Blauvelt (1990) discussed the issue of school security and recent litigation trends and stressed that security procedures and personnel must be system-wide decisions and cannot be left up to individual schools. Blauvelt made a number of recommendations:

- Schools need a uniform incident-reporting system to document security incidents.
- Schools must notify police when crimes occur.
- Security data need to be analyzed so that plans can be made to improve security.
- The school security department should be viewed as a specialized area in education and clearly defined with someone designated as Director of Security.
- Close communication must exist between the Superintendent and Director of Security.

Blauvelt pointed out that schools have five choices concerning security issues. They may:

1. Rely on local law enforcement.
2. Hire local police.
3. Contract with a guard service.
4. Hire security professionals.
5. Combination of 2, 3, and 4.

The school district that experiences little crime can rely solely on local law enforcement. A number of advantages and disadvantages are displayed in Table 4.4 for each of the options. It is apparent that much thought needs to be given to which option schools choose and that significant expenditures are needed for a good security or school police program.

Playground Safety

Bowers (1989) reported that 210,000 playground-related injuries were treated in hospital emergency rooms in 1987. There are many questions that arise about playground safety. It is obvious that injuries occur on the playground. The questions are how can we prevent playground injuries and manage playground incidents better? The following incident raises some of these questions:

TABLE 4.4. School Security Options: Advantages and Disadvantages

Options	Advantages	Disadvantages
1. Hire local police	Trained personnel Established reporting and communication procedures Clear authority Visibility high	Costly High turnover Don't report to school board May lack commitment to educational philosophy Lack of flexibility in dealing with students
2. Contract with guard service	Low cost Optional dress and weapon carrying School officials are in control of assignments, hiring, etc.	Not well trained School liability uncertain Lack of commitment to education High turnover Inadequate supervision
3. Hire security professionals	District does the hiring and decides role District determine dress and weapon issues In-house response for crisis Can design own reporting system	Must be budgeted in advance Costly May get involved in administrative and not just security issues Training program must be implemented

Note: Adapted from Blauvelt (1990).

A second-grade boy stepped behind a swing on the playground while another child was swinging. The boy was hit in the head and knocked unconscious. He later died. The principal became so agitated when she heard of the incident that she attempted to run across the playground in her high heels. She fell and broke her arm.

The first question is, how could this incident have been prevented? Closer supervision might have prevented it. A curriculum program on playground safety that had stressed never to run or walk behind swings might also have prevented it. Bowers points out two design issues that would have prevented this death.

1. Playgrounds should have physical barriers to discourage children from running into moving swings.
2. Swings should have soft seats instead of metal or wooden ones.

The principal in our example needed to control her emotional reaction and walk, not run, to the scene. If the principal had elected to run, she needed to remember to remove her high heels.

Bowers makes a number of recommendations for playground safety and points out that the traditional equipment is not very safe. Most injuries occur on swings, slides, and climbing equipment. Bowers called for designing equipment that minimizes the risk of injuries. Bowers made the following recommendations:

- Avoid steep slopes on playground equipment.
- Limit falls to 24 inches.
- Consider accessibility and allow children room to play on equipment at the same time (e.g., widen slides so that more than one child can go down at a time).
- Provide safe clearances by placing equipment at least 20 feet from trees, fences, etc.
- Install equipment in shady areas and minimize sun exposure.
- Use quality materials and inspect equipment regularly.
- Provide safe ground covering.
- Match equipment to ages of students.
- Increase playground supervision.

SUGGESTIONS TO DECREASE SCHOOL VIOLENCE

What is the cause of the violence in our schools? What can be done to reduce this violence? Harper (1989) reported the results of a teacher survey that listed the following causes of violence by school-aged children:

- Drug trafficking.
- Drug availability.
- Ease of access to guns.
- Lack of parental supervision.
- Lack of employment opportunities.

Muir (1988) reported some of the stretegies being used by the New York City schools to reduce violence. Those strategies included the following:

- Increase the number of security personnel.
- Assign security to after-school activities.
- Install two-way intercoms in every office.
- Provide secondary students with ID cards.
- Assign more police to arrival and dismissal times.
- Urge legislation to increase the penalty for crimes at school.

The National School Safety Center (NSSC) has made a number of additional recommendations to improve safety at school. Among their recommendations are the following:

1. Teach students to control their anger.
2. Provide law-related educational curriculum units.
3. Have adults highly visible in the halls and restrooms. Volunteers could be utilized.
4. Provide a safe-corridor program to assist students to get home safely.
5. Separate incompatible student groups.
6. Coordinate social work, delinquency, and at-risk programs.
7. Match potential student victims with a buddy to assist them.
8. Train the school staff in how to deescalate potentially violent situations.
9. Provide an anonymous reporting system to help stop violence and drug trafficking.
10. Promote antiweapon campaigns.
11. Provide reentry programs for those suspended and expelled.

The NSSC convened the superintendents from the nation's 15 largest school districts for what was termed the Urban School Safety Practicum. Several key strategies were suggested by those superintendents to help make schools safer:

1. Get the public more involved.
2. Improve school leadership.
3. Keep guns and weapons off campus.
4. Make school and neighborhoods drug-free.
5. Halt gang activity.
6. Increase youth discipline at home and at school.

These are a few of the many suggestions to reduce school violence. Perhaps the single, simplest recommendation for schools is to look at what is happening around them and at their school and to devote time and energy to confront the violence.

How Students Themselves Can Make Their School Safer

This question was addressed by Modglin (1989), who emphasized the importance of curriculum approaches. Modglin pointed out that students should have a vested interest in making school a safe place. Modglin commented, "Enlisting students in the crime prevention effort is not a panacea, but the result is safer and better schools, as well as students who have developed better interpersonal skills and increased sense of community and responsibility" (p. 10). Modglin makes the following suggestions as to how students can make their school safer:

1. Start a safe-watch program.
2. Allow older students to teach prevention information to younger students.
3. Provide mediation programs that help resolve disputes without violence.
4. Present prevention information to the student body.
5. Establish crime-prevention clubs to identify crime problems and develop strategies to reduce crime.
6. Promote community services projects to increase school pride.
7. Utilize student courts to dispose of student behavioral infractions.

These are all excellent ideas to involve students in helping prevent crisis situations. Our schools have begun programs such as the Safe-Ride Program to decrease drinking and driving and have conducted school crisis hotlines to help prevent youth suicide at the secondary level. Elementary schools have implemented programs to promote gun safety, bicycle safety, and seat-belt usage by students.

Environmental Design

Can we build safer schools? The answer from Ron Stevens, Director of the National School Safety Center, is yes! Stevens (1989) quoted the principal of the Greenwood, South Carolina school that experienced a shooting. The principal emphasized that school administrators must have visual access to maintain control and suggested a design like the spokes of a wheel so that administrators can view more of the school.

One Texas school (Huntsville) improved visual surveillance by placing cameras in the hallways and monitors in the administrative office.

A publication by the NSSC (1988) entitled *School Safety Checkbook* should be required reading for architectural firms and construction supervisors for school districts. One area discussed is called target hardening, and the following suggestions were made to reduce vandalism and violence and to increase safety.

- Locate schools in neighborhoods.
- Make entries visible.
- Limit roof access.
- Contain mechanical and electrical devices inside the school and have them locked up.
- Provide break-resistant exterior lights.
- Provide directional signs that indicate which way cars may enter.
- Build parking lots that are smaller and therefore safer and mix staff and students.
- Provide speed bumps to discourage cruising and reduce speed.
- Patrol grounds at night by police.
- Remove loose gravel around the school that could be thrown.
- Turn off all interior lights at night.
- Provide signs around the school that clearly state the rules for behavior.
- Provide parking areas with exit and entry gates.
- Remove exterior door handles from all but the front door.
- Trim shrubs so that no one can hide behind them.
- Start neighborhood watch programs to encourage the community to help monitor the school.
- Label school items that might be stolen with identification numbers.

Stevens (1989) indicated that schools in residential neighborhoods are the safest, and schools in general are five times more likely than businesses to be vandalized.

School architecture has recently begun to incorporate what is termed Crime Prevention Through Environmental Design (CPTED). This concept was discussed by Crowe (1990), who pointed out that the design and usage of school facilities has a direct relationship to code of conduct violations and criminal behavior. The most significant problem areas were the following.

- *School grounds* with overgrown shrubs, poorly defined borders, isolated areas, and bus loading near busy streets.

- *Parking lots* for students with multiple entrances and exits placed in remote areas on the campus periphery.
- *Locker rooms* with lockers assigned to more than one student; lockers with similar design and color that create confusion and decrease surveillance by making unclear transition zones; isolated lockers that invite theft.
- *Corridors* with "blind spots" that invite abnormal users. The least control in the school exists in the corridors.
- *Restrooms* are usually in isolated locations that present a perception of the area as "unsafe".
- *Classrooms* that are multipurpose do not promote responsibility and ownership for teachers and students.

Crowe made a number of recommendations to employ CPTED strategies to make school safer.

1. Locate gathering areas to where natural surveillance exists, and make gathering areas formal.
2. Reduce corridor congestion.
3. Provide clear borders for controlled space.
4. Personalize space to create ownership, and identify territories within the school.
5. Avoid large undifferentiated campuses.

These issues about environmental design are very important ones. The suggestion to make it difficult to gain access to the roof, for instance, caught our attention. Children have historically climbed on the school roofs. Sadly, in our district, two children fell through roof skylights and landed on the gym floor, suffering severe injury. Environmental design issues need to be examined and evaluated carefully.

What about Metal Detectors?

Piller (1990) reports that metal detectors are used in all Detroit city high schools and are used in a few New York City schools. Two types of metal detectors are used: hand-held and walk-through. Hand-held ones cost about $200, with walk-through ones being considerably more expensive. Only a small number of schools use metal detectors. Some that do use them report a decline in school violence. Many school districts, including the Houston city schools, have been debating whether or not to install them. Most school districts leave it up to the individual building principal to decide whether or not they are needed. The frequently voiced concerns about their usage are that guns and weapons will still get in and administrators, teachers, parents, and students don't like the image that having metal detectors portrays. The decision of whether or not to install metal detectors is a difficult one. Our recommendation is that all schools have available a portable one.

Guns and the Schools

"Carrying weapons has become an acceptable risk for too many students. The presence of weapons on campus places the entire academic community at risk and makes everyone a potential victim" (*Weapons in Schools*, 1990, p. 12). Estimates are that at least 100,000 school children carry a gun to school each day in this country. Surveys of students have shown that most can get a gun if they want to, and most know someone who has brought a gun to school.

The debate about guns and gun control has raged for decades in this country. Guns are a problem in our society and represent a very real problem and threat to the safety of our schools. One of the administrators in our school district, Bill Martin, commented, "I have been in education 24 years and guns were involved in every serious crisis I faced as an administrator except one."

A recent article in *USA Today*, Waiting Period Can Curb Handgun Toll (1990), gave the following facts about guns in the United States:

- Every 2½ minutes someone is injured with a gun.
- A teen commits suicide with a gun every 3 hours.
- Every day a child is killed by a gun.
- Every year 30,000 people are murdered with a gun.
- Every year 12,000 people commit suicide with a gun.
- Every year 1,500 Americans are killed in accidents with guns.
- Sixty million Americans own guns.

Sperling (1990) points out that the murder rate for young men in the United States is four times that of any other developed country. Keen (1989) emphasized that weapons are used in 70,000 assaults in schools each year. A *USA Today* article, "One Day in the Lives of U.S.A. Children" (1990) reported that 30 children are wounded by guns daily.

A resource paper, *Weapons in Schools* (1990), published by the National School Safety Center contained the following facts and figures:

- 1,000 homicide victims under the age of 19 are killed by guns each year.

- 3,000 youths annually commit suicide with a firearm.
- Knives are the most common weapon brought to school, but sophisticated firearms are readily available to students.
- Kids carry guns to school to show off, because they fear for their safety, or because violence is part of our society.
- Guns at school are related to drug trafficking in the community.
- Guns are contained in every other household and may total 120 million.

Time published an article entitled, "Shootouts in the Schools" (1989). The article quoted a teacher who faced a kindergartener with a gun who said, "Whatever is out on the streets seeps into the schools" (p. 116). The article pointed out that over 100,000 children carry a gun to school each day and that schools face legal liability if they have not taken steps to prepare for this. The article outlines the following strategies that educators have tried to cope with gun violence at school:

- Increase security personnel.
- Install metal detectors.
- Require students to have ID cards.
- Give cash awards to students who report potential violence.
- Train school staff in emergency procedures.
- Conduct bullet drills that teach students to hit the deck when bullets fly.
- Build walls around schools.

The National School Safety Center's resource paper on *Weapons in Schools* also discussed intervention strategies. The paper emphasized that no national figures are kept on gun deaths at school. There are clippings with horrifying headlines and maps pinpointing the various locations around the country. It seems clear that 43,500 gun deaths a year will affect almost all of the 93,000 schools in this country sooner or later. One can conclude that gun deaths, guns brought to school, and school violence are at an all-time high. The following additional strategies have been tried by the schools according to the NSSC:

- Set a clear school policy with regard to weapon violation with swift suspension or expulsion.
- Make it difficult for students to conceal a weapon by requiring open lockers and mesh book bags.
- Have reentry programs and counseling programs for students caught with weapons.
- Establish school security committees.

- Limit access to school grounds.
- Teach students to take responsibility for school safety and report suspicious individuals and unusual activity.
- Have students sign nonviolence contracts.
- Increase public awareness that "guns kill."
- Implement violence prevention units in the curriculum.
- Introduce curriculum units on gun safety.

It seems clear that getting the parents involved is important if we are to reduce the number of guns that are brought to school. One school locally tried just such a strategy. Parents of all 2,300 students at the high school were invited to attend a meeting to discuss the large number of pistols being brought to school. Moran (1990) reported that only 36 parents showed up and that school officials were frustrated by the lack of response on the part of the parents.

Dade County, Florida schools have implemented a curriculum program designed to reduce handgun deaths. A review of the program shows that there is hope that handgun deaths will be reduced by the following:

1. Providing information to students grades K through 12 about the danger of guns.
2. Letting students hear from victims themselves about the danger of guns.
3. Providing legal information about the consequences of not safeguarding guns from children.

It is interesting to note that the Dade County program is repeated three times in each school each year. Most school presentations are given one time only. The program does not teach children how to handle guns but, instead, emphasizes that children are to stay away from guns. The program also involves parent meetings, public service messages on radio and television, and brochures on gun safety, ownership, storage, and usage. A poster depicts the overall theme of the program: "Guns Kill, Say No to Guns!" The reverse side of the poster contains famous last words:

"I didn't know it was loaded."
"I thought it was a toy."
"I was angry for just a moment."

The Dade County program looks very promising. It is important that all children be taught to be careful around guns and to report guns to adults. The program also emphasizes the landmark legislation that was passed by the Florida legislature in 1989. The law, entitled "Florida Kids and Guns Law," holds adults responsible for safeguarding guns from children under age 16. It is a felony in Florida to cause injury to a minor by storing or leaving a loaded firearm within reach or easy access to a minor. Snider (1990) cited research estimating that 1 million latchkey children go home to a house where there is a gun. Poland (1989a) quoted the suicide note left behind by a teen-age suicide victim who asked her parents why they made it so easy for her to kill herself by leaving a gun available to her.

Guns are a threat to the safety of everyone at school. Efforts must be continued to keep guns off campus. Metal detectors alone are not the answer, although schools should have access to portable hand-held metal detectors. The entire school community including school personnel, parents, and, most of all, the students themselves need to keep guns off campus. If a gun is on campus, students always know it—the critical question is, did any student come forward and alert security or administrative personnel? Gun deaths and murders are at an all-time high according to Kell (1990), and 12% of all homicide arrests are for children under 18 years of age. Wolf (1991) reported that handguns account for 48% of all murders in this country and that handguns comprise 70 million of the 200 million guns now in the country. In addition two million handguns are made each year in the U.S.A. Curriculum units must deal with the societal problems of guns. Perhaps a future generation of Americans will choose not to have a gun in every other home.

Bomb Threats

What should be done to deal with bomb threats at school? There needs to be a well-thought-out district or school policy. Most school administrators are faced with the decision of whether or not to evacuate the school. Most of the time school is evacuated, and a "lucky group" of school personnel search for the bomb before school is resumed. We do not have the answers, but we are aware that many school districts are not pleased with their policy in this area.

The principal of the school answered the phone 5 minutes before the bell was to ring to dismiss school for Christmas vacation. The principal panicked when the caller said a bomb was going to go off and hung up. The principal immediately grabbed the public address microphone and announced throughout the large school, without even introducing himself, "Everybody out now, the school is going to blow up!" The students and faculty were very unsure of what to do, and many students refused to leave school without first getting their personal belongings.

The question of whether or not to evacuate the school will always remain a judgment call for school officials. School officials must avoid panicking. Policies to handle bomb threats, need to be reviewed and discussed. In particular, schools can do something about bomb threats: They can utilize a standardized reporting form like the one developed by the National School Safety Center (1988). The form needs to be kept in the main office and be accessible to the switchboard operator. The form encourages the person answering the 'phone to stay calm and gather informaion from the caller, including the following:

1. Where is the bomb?
2. What kind is it?
3. When will it go off?
4. Why have you planted it?
5. Who are you?

In addition, the form has a checklist for characteristics of the caller and background noises. A careful gathering of such information will be very helpful to guide the administrator and to aid the police in tracing and apprehending the caller. Schools also can set up a tape recorder to record incoming calls to help catch the perpetrators of bomb threats.

Teacher Victimization

Feder (1989) discussed the efforts in the New York City schools to support teachers who are the victims of violence. She gave numerous examples of teachers who felt ignored and unsupported after having been victims of violence. In one case, police left a teacher alone in the same room with the student who had just attacked her. Teachers are often asked to take themselves to the hospital following the violent incident. Other victimized teachers reported that when they had returned to school the principal did not look them in the eyes or welcome them back.

Feder stressed that administrators must provide immediate and ongoing support to help the victim. She made the following points:

- The victims need clear and accurate information about work procedures, paperwork, benefits, and legal rights.
- The victims need to have their feelings validated and need an opportunity to talk about the incident and their feelings that they were somehow to blame.
- The victims are very needy of support and may perceive no support when it is seen as being offered by the administrator.

Feder pointed out that administrators may want to focus on the victims themselves and how they "contributed" to the incident rather than to focus on the fact that something is very wrong with the system when teachers are getting attacked. Administrators may ignore or minimize the very natural feelings of fear and rage that these victims experience.

The question of what teacher gets attacked was also addressed by Feder. Feder found that teacher victims were characterized by the following:

- Minority status.
- Authoritative or elitist style.
- Personal or professional insecurity.
- A history of victimization.

There needs to be more emphasis on how schools can prevent teacher victimization. Glenn (1990) suggested that school personnel can protect themselves by:

- Avoiding solitude and isolation.
- Doing things in groups.
- Discussing safety issues with administrators and community members and devising procedures to make school safer.

Teachers who have been victimized need ongoing support and a careful reentry program to school.

Gangs

The number of youth gangs in this country is on the increase. Gangs are more mobile than ever before and have reached suburban and rural areas. Crime is the common threat in gang activity, and it ranges from mischief to drug sales and drive-by shootings (Moran, 1991). Gangs are dramatically affecting our schools.

What is the role of the schools with regard to gangs? What impact can gangs have on the climate of a school? What resources are available to help the schools to prevent gang activity? Muck (1991) emphasized that the best source of information about gangs is the school. Muck stressed that schools must admit when they have a gang problem and keep in close contact with police agencies.

The reasons young people join gangs are complex, with no simple answer; however, Horswell (1991) stressed that many members joined out of a need for belonging. Harper (1989) cited the following reasons for gang membership: protection, acceptance, excitement, monetary gain, peer pressure, and few alternatives besides membership. Garrison (1989) pointed out that gangs often recruit juveniles because the legal penalities for criminal acts committed by juveniles are less severe. Muck (1990) reported that Texas has proposed legislation to increase penalties for criminal behavior related to gang activity.

What are the signs of gang activity that parents and school personnel can look for in a particular child? The following signs were listed by Horswell (1991):

1. Dressing the same each day and insisting on certain clothes or accessories.
2. Body tattoos or graffiti on personal belongings.
3. Drop in school performance and attendance.
4. Discipline problems, drinking, or drug abuse.
5. Change of friends and social activities.
6. Unexplained increase in money and personal items.
7. Late hours.

Much has been written about the role of the schools with regard to prevention and intervention with gangs. The National School Safety Center has written a manual entitled, *Gangs in Schools: Breaking Up Is Hard to Do* (National School Safety Center, 1990). The manual outlined numerous strategies for the schools and stressed the following:

1. Enforce behavior codes firmly and consistently.
2. Photograph gang graffiti for criminal prosecution and then remove it promptly.
3. Identify gang members on campus and confer with them.
4. Keep all schools neutral territory.
5. In-service staff members about gangs.
6. Increase security personnel.
7. Offer parenting and counseling programs to divert gang involvement.
8. Share information with other schools and all state and law enforcement agencies to suppress gang activity.
9. Eliminate confrontation between gangs and intimidation of students.

Many school systems have begun to learn about gangs and are making efforts to decrease gang activities in the schools. We must recognize that gangs are a threat to the safety and security of our schools.

5

When Crisis Affects a Community Preparing for School-Wide Crisis or Disaster

COCONUT GROVE, BUFFALO CREEK, AND THREE MILE ISLAND: WHAT LESSONS CAN BE LEARNED FROM COMMUNITY DISASTERS?

Unraveling the problem of helping large numbers of individuals in crisis has been a topic of research and discussion for most of the 20th century. Some of the original thinking has been discarded; other ideas have stood the test of time. Many of the trends and policies documented in community disasters transfer very clearly to school community disasters or school-wide building crises. Crises such as shootings, food poisonings, multiple deaths, and bus accidents produce large groups of emotional, bereaved, and sometimes panic-stricken individuals. What is a district or a school psychologist to do in the face of events that seem to overwhelm the routine mental health resources? This is the question we attempt to answer in this chapter. The solutions are based in part on past research and documentation of disaster cases in communities and schools together with our 10 years of experience in managing such crises in the schools.

Traditionally, the psychological and emotional elements in disastrous events were not areas of concern or focus. Until the 1970s, intervention in disasters focused almost entirely on the delivery of services to meet physical needs: food, clothing, shelter, and rebuilding. Despite the widespread belief that such shocks might engender severe psychopathology, psychological first aid was given little attention (Taylor, Ross, &

Quarantelli, 1976). Over the years, however, a few modern disasters have received careful study and become hallmark cases in disaster-related mental health intervention. They include the Coconut Grove fire (Lindemann, 1944), the Buffalo Creek flood (Titchener & Kapp, 1976), and the Chowchilla kidnappings (Terr, 1983).

In 1974 a Federal Disaster Law was passed mandating that "training and services in relief of mental health problems in major disasters" should also be provided. More recent studies springboard from this law and focus on psychological needs as well as others, for example, the stress-response syndrome following the Mount St. Helens eruption (Shore, Tatum, & Vollmer, 1986), and posttraumatic stress among Cambodian refugees (Kinzee, 1986).

Overall, studies suggest that significant mental health problems did arise in the aftermath of such crisis events. However, researchers also appear to be reaching the general consensus that serious mental illness or severe, sustained psychiatric disturbance do not result from a singular exposure to a disaster (Auerbach & Spirito, 1986; Tuckman, 1973; Schulberg, 1974; Zarle, Hartsough, & Ottinger, 1974; Kirn, 1975; Heffron, 1975; Taylor et al., 1976; Frederick, 1977), although some controversy continues to exist (Shore, 1986).

Somewhat surprisingly, there is typically an absence of demand for traditional mental health services; some chronic psychiatrically troubled individuals may even improve their functioning as they rally to avoid potential physical devastation. Responses reported by communities following a disaster are most commonly at least temporarily positive and altruistic: sharing of private property, dissolution of normal social barriers, and readiness to take unknown victims into homes (Dynes, 1978; Prince, 1920; Perry & Perry, 1959; Perry, Silber, & Bloch, 1956). Contrary to what the media might have us believe, rioting, looting, and panic are rarely recorded following natural disasters (Chapman, 1962; Taylor et al., 1976).

Traditional psychotherapy needs following disasters do not appear to be as significant as those for crisis intervention. As in individual crisis intervention, researchers report "normal, healthy" people experiencing temporary emotional difficulty caused by losses and stress. It is therefore generally recommended that postdisaster mental health services be built around a social service delivery model because most disaster-related problems tend to be temporary "problems in living" that do not significantly threaten day-to-day social performance.

There is, however, some suggestion that crises or disasters associated with the actions of humans are more traumatic and difficult to recover from than those generated by natural events (Lifton & Olson, 1976). Aggression and deliberate maliciousness seem to strike hardest into our

Preparing for Disaster

psyche. Such patterns have been noted among the children and families
of concentration camp survivors (Rakoff, 1966).

Most often the recommended social services model provides social
support services by voluntary groups and agencies staffed by nonprofes-
sionals. It must be acknowledged, however, that there remain many
unanswered questions regarding specific psychological needs following
disasters (Smith, 1989).

Professionals and paraprofessionals in schools do appear to be key
individuals for supporting the community in a natural disaster, man-
made disaster, or school-district disaster. Under such circumstances, it is
easy to put the school in a crisis-interventionist role, for school personnel
have historically found themselves involved in supporting community
problems in diverse ways. The schools find themselves providing food,
clothing, and shelter, providing mediation in angry family disputes,
caring for issues and concerns regarding children's reactions, etc.

Three other themes emerge from accounts of those providing mental
health services in disasters that are also pertinent to the functioning of
the school in the community (Tierney & Baisden, 1979, p. 42):

1. The sense is that victims require support services *where they are*
   rather than in a hospital or mental health clinic.
2. Mental health providers are often most needed to act as resources
   for access to other community services and thus must be well
   informed regarding the diversity of services available. A very large
   part of the mental health effort in the above mentioned crises
   involved putting individuals in touch with needed services, even to
   the point of physically getting them there.
3. The use of paraprofessionals and volunteers provides a vital service, especially when those individuals are already known as helpful resources in the community.

Special-Needs Populations

Although there is little solid research that indicates that some groups of
individuals react differently to disasters, mental health services have
attempted to focus on groups believed to require special attention.
These groups almost always include children. Several studies were
made, and the services offered were most frequently for the purpose of
reducing the children's disaster-related fears (Howard & Gordon, 1972).
Other hypothetical target groups are families who have lost one or more
loved ones; those who have lost their homes and have to relocate; and
those experiencing serious economic loss because of the disaster.

Stages in the Appearance of Disaster-Related Mental Health Needs

Many theorists have broken disasters into stages for conceptual clarity and for the purpose of organizing a plan of action. The stages vary in number and content. Dynes (1974), for example, suggests eight time stages: predisaster conditions, warning, threat, impact, inventory, rescue, remedy, and recovery. Differential involvement of various community organizations is suggested at each stage. Barton (1970) distinguishes fewer stages: the predisaster period, the detection and warning period, the period of immediate response, the period of organized social response, and the long-run postdisaster period.

The overarching theme is that many community members will experience the same types of need at roughly the same period of time. Table 5.1 provides the essential ideas at a glance.

Factors Affecting Recovery

Although present research suggests that the prevalence and severity of severe psychopathology have probably been overestimated, varying degrees of social disruption may require professional attention.

A number of researchers have attempted to examine the outstanding features of community or school disasters to determine which characteristics shock people the most (Tyhurst, 1951). It appears that reaction and recovery are influenced by several factors. Below is a summary of current thought, which certainly is still evolving and under speculation:

1. The proportion of the involved population. This is apparently more of a factor than the exact numbers of individuals affected (Baum, Fleming, & Davidson, 1983).

2. The element of surprise (predictability) of the incident. If and when warnings are given, they should be followed by instructions of what to do. Warning followed by long silences and no action plan can heighten anxiety and lead to the commonly observed denial that a disaster is imminent. Disaster recurrence often has the effect of "quasiroutinizing" disaster, making it less disruptive and disturbing.

3. Familiarity. Crisis or disaster affects individuals inasmuch as it provides disturbing experiences with which children and adults are unfamiliar. Such experiences including seeing or handling the dead (Hershiser & Quarantelli, 1976; Blanshan, 1977; Blanshan & Quarantelli, 1981) and seeing badly injured or disfigured individuals seem to

TABLE 5.1. Postcrisis Needs of Victims of Disaster

Help needed	Possible outcomes if help is unavailable
Phase I: Impact (immediately) Information on source and degree of danger Escape and rescue from immediate source of danger Locate loved ones Chance for ventilation	Physical injury or death Severe stress reactions
Phase II: Recoil (days/weeks later) Shelter, food, drink, clothing, medical care Support for coping with exhaustion, frustration, and discouragement	Physical injury Delayed grief reactions
Phase III: Posttraumatic (months to a year later) Physical reconstruction Social reestablishment Psychological support concerning aftermath effects of event: aftermath effects of the event itself; bereavement counseling concerning loss of loved ones, home, and personal property	Financial hardship Social instability Longer-lasting adjustment problems

Note. Adapted from Hoff (1978), p. 232.

interfere with coping abilities. Thus, individuals who witness these events and are first-hand responders may not be the ones to provide ongoing support.

4. Separation of family members. Children are particularly vulnerable to damaging psychological effects if separated from their family during the acute period of a disaster (Blanford & Levine, 1972). Therefore, families should generally be kept together, and shocked children returned to their parents as soon as is practical.

5. Outside help. Reasonable recovery from a physical disaster demands that aid must be provided from areas not affected by the disaster. Often military forces are called in. Individuals providing emotional

support for adults and children may likewise need to be "imported" from a nearby location.

6. Leadership. As in any crisis situation, a disaster demands that someone have the ability to make decisions and give direction. In the community, the police, the military, and physicians have "built-in" potential for leadership during a disaster. Leadership in the schools is less clear, but certainly district administrators should be among those ready to "call the shots" in the case of a school-district disaster.

7. Communication. Since failures in communication give rise to rumors, it is essential that a communication network and public information centers be established and maintained. Much impulsive and irrational behavior can be prevented by the reassurance and direction that a good communication network provides.

8. Measures directed toward reorientation. Communication lays the foundation for the reidentification of individuals in family and social groups. A basic step in reorientation is the opportunity to locate and discuss the incident with fellow victims so that they can once again feel like members of the school society.

9. Evacuation of populations. In any disaster there is a spontaneous mass movement to leave the stricken area. Planned evacuation will prevent panic, especially if escape is blocked and delayed. A failure to attend to the psychological and social problems of evacuation can result in serious social and interpersonal problems.

10. The length of involvement in a crisis. Some kind of threshold or breaking point is reached if the crisis continues, unabated, for a long enough period. Exactly what this length of time is is difficult to specify.

Childhood Reactions to Community/School Disasters

There is a reasonable body of research that suggests that a fair percentage of children exposed to natural disasters will experience "circumscribed, time-limited fears or behavioral problems" (Auerbach & Spirito, 1986, p. 194). Further, those who were most directly involved with the event, the immediate parent reactions, and family and community support following the disaster appeared to affect this reaction.

Children overall appear to react to calamity with (1) increased anxiety regarding separation from family and loved ones and (2) some age-related regression (Farberow & Gordon, 1981). Recommendations in the treatment of stress related to disasters include the following.

1. As in all crisis counseling, remember that victims view themselves as anxious and under stress but not as pathological.
2. Children separated from their parents and family during a disaster

will need a great deal of comforting and reassurance during the interim. News regarding the whereabouts and safety of their family, phone calls from parents, etc., should be provided as soon as possible.

3. The family should be considered the first line of assistance for helping children to adjust to the disaster. This is true in regard to promoting a faster adjustment. Benedek (1979) reviewed the literature in this area and concluded that a stable and caring parent was probably the most essential element in the child's adjustment to catastrophe. Other researchers (Raphael, 1975) concluded that maintaining close family ties, reassurance, and open discussion are the most important elements.

4. Disaster treatment and services in general mandate that professionals working with the disaster situation seek out potential beneficiaries instead of waiting for victims to seek help. Tuckman (1973) noted that reaching out immediately to disaster victims and families during a crisis can prevent the development of posttraumatic symptoms. This particular aspect of disaster is what often intimately involves schools in community assistance projects not necessarily related to education or even occurring during the course of the school day. Schools are frequently used as disaster assistance centers to provide services on site, information on the availability of community services, or consultation to parents and children. School staff may be asked to interface with a community mental disaster team in order to attain these goals.

5. School-aged victims of disaster should be encouraged to participate in daily activities that provide emotional support and help the child to develop a realistic appraisal of the situation and to confront it. In addition, these activities provide opportunities for personal expression regarding the crisis event (Crabbs, 1981).

The National Institute of Mental Health, similarly, makes three key recommendations when a crisis involves children:

1. Remember that children are resilient.
2. Work with the child and his or her parents if possible. The flight attendant on an airplane tells us that if we are traveling with a small child and the cabin loses oxygen, we should reach up and get the oxygen mask and place it over our mouth first and then the child's next. This analogy points out the need for working with parents first.
3. Mental health personnel should seek out those who need their help. We cannot sit in our offices and wait for the victims of a crisis to seek us out. Mental health personnel should be highly visible in the schools following a crisis.

CHOWCHILLA, COKEVILLE, CONCORD, WINNETKA, GREENWOOD, AND STOCKTON: WHAT LESSONS CAN BE LEARNED FROM SCHOOL-DISTRICT DISASTERS?

Major crisis events for the schools occurred in the above locations, spanning a 20-year period. What has been learned from these events? How can the schools be prepared to prevent and manage crisis situations? Have the schools improved their ability to manage crisis situations? There is considerable evidence that the volume of crisis situations and violence that occur in schools have increased. One could reach the conclusion that any catastrophic event that can be imagined has already happened at a school somewhere in this country. We have saved hundreds of newspaper headlines that deal with school crises and have read a few of them to get the attention of school administrators at the beginning of an in-service designed to motivate them to organize a crisis team. One participant commented, "I wanted you to stop reading those horrible headlines depicting violence, but then I remembered the audience and thought, no, to reach this group—he'd better read them all!"

Chowchilla, California

An incident that is so horrible that it is hard to believe it really happened occurred in Chowchilla, California in the early 1970s. A busload of children grades K–12 was kidnaped and buried in the desert for 3 days. The kidnapers had dug a hole, driven the bus in, and then covered it. The children dug their way out and escaped. They were physically unhurt but were, or course, tired and hungry. Sandall (1986) has discussed this incident in depth. The children were told to go home and forget about the incident. Terr (1983) found that 5 years later 100% of the Chowchilla children had clinical symptoms of depression, anxiety, or fears about the world. A number of the Chowchilla children, who are now adults, have appeared on television and discussed their experience. They report problems in their adult lives as a result of this incident. The response of the Chowchilla schools and the local mental health officials follows only one of the National Institute of Mental Health principles for working with children after disaster, and that is that children are resilient. These victims were not provided with immediate counseling at school or at the mental health center. A teacher who had lived in Chowchilla at that time commented to us that it is an affluent area, and it was believed that parents would seek out the needed psychological assistance for their children.

Cokeville, Wyoming

In May of 1986 a couple entered Cokeville Elementary School and took 160 adults and children hostage. The couple demanded ransom money to finance a revolution. Accidentally discharging a bomb they had used to threaten the hostages, the couple was killed, and 80 adults and children were injured. Sandall (1986) discussed the crisis intervention efforts to assist the students and faculty of the elementary school. Sandall, the school psychologist for the district, was designated as the crisis coordinator. Sandall and the principal decided that an immediate and active response was required. The following are a few of the actions taken:

1. A town meeting was held the next day, a Saturday. The meeting assisted students, their families, and the community to cope with the crisis.
2. Children were encouraged to visit the school as soon as possible.
3. Faculty meetings were held to discuss the incident and how to assist the students.
4. Students were encouraged to discuss the incident and their feelings fully. Feelings were expressed through discussion, writing, and artwork.
5. School was resumed as soon as possible with numerous opportunities for discussion of the incident provided.

Sandall found that the children who verbalized in the greatest quantity and those who attended school the most after the incident managed to recover the best. Those children who were having difficulty recovering were provided long-term assistance and were encouraged to attend summer school. Stevens (1989) discussed the Cokeville incident and the active response of the school; he emphasized that the crisis intervention policy now in place in Cokeville is extremely comprehensive.

Concord, New Hampshire

Christa McAuliffe was a teacher at Concord High School. Schulman (1986) discussed what steps were taken to assist the students and faculty to cope with the space shuttle disaster that killed Christa McAuliffe and the other astronauts. The school had already experienced a hostage situation a month earlier that had resulted in death. A crisis team had been formed as a result of that previous incident, and Schulman stressed that the crisis team was prepared to manage the death of Christa Mc-Auliffe without the outside assistance that was offered. Students were encouraged to stay at school as long as needed on the day of the disaster to talk out their feelings. School was dismissed for only one day. When school resumed students were given several choices besides attending class. They could vent frustration and anger through physical activity in the gym, or they could congregate in the cafeteria to receive group support. Those students who wished to be alone with their thoughts could go to the library, which served as a quiet area. Schulman stressed the importance of having a trained crisis team in the schools and stressed that the resolution of the second tragedy helped resolve leftover feelings from the earlier one.

Winnetka, Illinois

In May 1988, a 30-year-old woman walked into Hubbards Woods Elementary School in Winnetka, Illinois and shot six students. The woman then killed herself. "The shootings have forever changed the fabric of our affluent community," said Harry Dillard, the head of psychological services for the school district, speaking on a panel at a national workshop (Dillard, 1990). Dillard discussed his initial response to the shootings that took the life of the son of a school board member. He commented that the administration of the school system had discouraged him from going to the scene of the shooting. Dillard took his staff and went to the school. He described his initial thoughts as wondering if he would need to provide first aid. Instead, he found that psychological first aid was what he needed to provide (Dillard, 1989).

Dillard and his staff went from classroom to classroom seeking out those children who needed assistance. Children were given the facts about what had happened and were encouraged to express their emotions. Dillard pointed out that reading the book *Alexander's No Good Day,* written by Judith Viorst, helped children express their emotions. Dillard described the posttraumatic stress disorder experienced by many of the children and adults at Hubbards Woods School. Plans were developed that outlined both short-term and long-term activities to help reduce the effects of the crisis. Parent and community meetings were held. Mental health professionals from outside the school were utilized. Parents and children were provided with counseling services over the summer to help them resolve the incident. Follow-up efforts continued during the next school year.

Dillard pointed out that when the Stockton, California shooting occurred the following January, there was a need to meet again with faculty and parents. A number of parents expressed the desire at that time to build a wall around the school and the playground and to hire armed guards for the hallways. Dillard, in reviewing the incident and the parents' responses, made these suggestions for other school districts:

1. Establish close cooperative relations with the fire department and police in your community.
2. Be familiar with the mental health resources available to assist you.
3. Provide clear, direct, and honest communication about the incident to all concerned.
4. Keep the school open for information and counseling.
5. Provide counseling opportunities for children and their parents.
6. Use group meetings to convey factual information and dispel rumors.
7. Help the faculty to understand posttraumatic stress, what to expect from the children, and how to help both the children and themselves.
8. Develop plans for the anniversary reaction.

Dillard (1990) provided an overview of how parents and children were coping 8 months after the incident. The majority of the children reported that they were still scared (93%), and 70% reported that they were experiencing bad dreams. Fifty percent of the parents surveyed reported that they felt less able to protect their children after the incident. Dillard stressed that counseling the victims in the first 24 hours is essential and that those children who had cohesive family units recovered most quickly.

Greenwood, South Carolina

A gunman named Jamie Wilson wounded nine and killed two at Oakland Elementary School in Greenwood, South Carolina on September 26, 1988. Greer (1988) interviewed Wilson after the shooting and reported that he had been influenced by the Winnetka shootings and other violence in our society as well as his own negative memories of public school. There is little information available on the management of this incident. Stevens (1989) reported that the custodian of the elementary school saw Wilson enter the building dressed in camouflage clothing with a rifle over his shoulder. The custodian reportedly waved at Wilson and went on with his custodial work. This incident illustrates the following key point: Everyone must be alert, and all school employees must be trained in crisis intervention.

If the custodian had alerted the principal and/or authorities, perhaps some or all of the deaths or injuries could have been prevented.

Stockton, California

The most violent incident ever to occur on school grounds happened on January 17, 1989 at Cleveland Elementary School in Stockton. Busher

(1990) reported that a gunman named Patrick Purdy fired an estimated 105 rounds in less than 2 minutes from an AK-47 assault rifle at students and teachers on the playground. The gunman was dressed in camouflage clothing and fired from two different locations. The students and teachers initially thought that firecrackers were going off. Five students were killed, and 29 students and a teacher were injured. The gunman committed suicide when police arrived on the scene. Busher complimented the Stockton emergency medical response and reported that all victims were at the hospital in less than 1 hour. Busher stressed that the Stockton paramedics and fire department routinely rehearsed their response to medical emergencies. It was initially feared that 10 of the wounded would not survive, but they all did. Busher in reviewing this incident made the following points:

- Crisis drills practiced monthly at the school undoubtedly saved lives.
- Problems were immediately encountered in identifying the dead and wounded.
- Language barriers existed to communicating with the parents of the students, as most of the families were from Southeast Asia.
- Fifty mental health workers came to the school the evening of the shooting to assist, and these workers were available for individual classrooms when shool opened the next day.
- A faculty meeting was held the next day that gave teachers a choice of whether or not to utilize a mental health worker in their classes.
- School personnel were assigned to work with the families of the wounded and deceased.

Armstrong (1990b), the school psychologist assigned to the school, also discussed the incident and emphasized the following initial problems and concerns:

- Crowd control was a problem and needs to be a part of crisis planning.
- Educators were divided on the issue of whether or not it was important for the students to talk about their fears and emotions after the incident.
- Many victims had religious beliefs that pain should be borne in silence.
- Southeast Asian community members thought the incident was racially motivated.
- Rumors persisted that there was more than one gunman.
- Fear and rumors probably accounted for only 250 of 970 students coming to school the next day.
- Crisis workers were not prepared for the posttraumatic stress reaction experienced by most students.

- School staff went out into the community to encourage parents to send their children back to school.
- Many school staff members were reluctant to talk about their own emotions, and, in particular, the staff wanted their debriefing and processing to occur during school hours.

Armstrong was very active in advocating counseling for the students at the school. He commented that 3 weeks after the incident he alone was left to provide counseling to the victims. He had a list of over 300 students whom he was concerned about. Armstrong (1990a) reported that the students who verbalized the most and those who spoke to a counselor in their native language recovered the best. He also reported that the school district administration underestimated what was needed to assist students though this crisis. Teachers marched on the central office and demanded more counseling for the students. This action, and the media coverage of it, prompted the central office to provide more counselors to the school. More counseling assistance was located, and a team of psychologists and counselors from Winnetka, Illinois flew in to assist.

Armstrong pointed out that some resistance should be expected in every tragedy and that a crisis will exacerbate existing problems in the community. In this case many of the problems involved cultural differences between the Southeast Asian families and others in the community. Cultural differences resulted in debate about exactly what steps needed to be taken to resolve the crisis. Most of the families of the victims were Buddhists, and several exorcisms were conducted on school grounds to remove evil spirits. Two months after the incident, the St. Patrick's Day parade added to the cultural difficulties. Initially, the Southeast Asian families were confused and thought the gunman, Patrick Purdy, was being honored with a parade.

Armstrong (1990b) stressed that counseling be continued throughout the summer for students and that school be the source of the healing. The response of the school district was an active one, but it was necessary for Armstrong and others to advocate strongly for more counseling help for students. Armstrong also raised the question of what if this incident had occurred in a rural area instead of a city? Where would the additional counselors have come from? This incident also points out the need for school administrators to know their community and, in particular, to make plans to manage cultural differences when a crisis occurs.

There have been many articles in school administration journals in the last few years about crises. These articles are usually written in the first person and have headlines that emphasize the terror, uncertainty, and confusion that the administrator felt. The articles are written to try to help other administrators to be prepared; headlines emphasize that "forewarned is forearmed." We have provided in-services on this subject all over the country and have found that there are skeletons in the closet everywhere. All schools have experienced crisis situations, and many school employees wish they had somehow done something different to manage or prevent the crisis. There is not enough emphasis on preparation for the future.

There is considerable evidence that schools will continue to face severe crisis situations. What can be done? How can they be better prepared? What can be learned from the tragedies that have already occurred?

TERTIARY PREVENTION: THE SCHOOL'S FIRST BUILDING CRISIS

School psychologists and administrators frequently are looked to as the most appropriate personnel to intervene and support the schools in times of crisis. In inexperienced or unprepared districts, however, a call for help usually is made at what is (interventionwise) the least advantageous moment: shortly after the crisis has occurred. The crisis may represent a situation for which there has been no preparation. The school district is, in effect, "caught with its plans down." In case examples of this sort a predictable profile of problems begins to emerge. Through the following example you may witness this phenomenon for yourself.

In the next few pages, a real life disaster that occurred in a district without specific crisis intervention plans is summarized. The response to this shooting was an example of what Oates (1988) terms a spontaneous response in emphasizing that schools basically have three reactions to a crisis situation:

1. Ignore it.
2. Respond spontaneously.
3. Respond based on preplanning.

The third option is certainly the best. Our school district simply wasn't prepared to respond based on prior planning. Nor could a situation this extreme be ignored. All in all, the response that the elementary school and the district made under very trying conditions was very commendable.

Case Study: Face to Face with Disaster

"A student has been shot while raising the flag in front of an elementary school, and students at a junior high school have been fired upon." We will never forget hearing those words, as one of us had a son who went to school in the area where the shooting had taken place. As a professional, his thoughts, however, had to be focused on services to the school. We were uncertain as to what we could do to help but felt a need to go to the schools. One psychologist tried to excuse himself from the special education committee meeting and was told that he definitely was needed there. When we indicated that we felt a crisis took priority over planning to meet the I.E.P. needs of a special education student, we were told that we could assist with the crisis later. It was annoying that the immediacy of the response should be curtailed by routine special education meetings.

We were apprehensive about being at the scene of the shooting and were unsure about what services could even be offered. Attempts to call the school where the boy had been shot all failed. A reporter from the local television station called and requested an interview. The reporter wanted to focus on how parents could help their children cope with this crisis. We felt sure that the superintendent's office would handle all interviews and directed the reporter to call that office. The phone rang again, and this time it was the superintendent, who indicated that psychological services should grant the interview in accordance with current policy of cooperating with interview requests from the media.

None of us had ever done a television interview, and we knew nothing about the media policies of the school district. Our attempts at passing the buck had failed. What should be said? Psychology staff who were in the office were consulted in the few minutes it would take the camera crew to arrive. Suggestions were made: be brief and direct; emphasize that parents need to control their own reactions and focus on their children's emotions; try to be a calming influence; recommend letting the child talk about his or her concerns; make the point that adults need to model being in control and that steps have been taken by school administrators to gain control over the crisis situation. We rehearsed these points aloud while waiting to be interviewed.

As the television reporter explained his objectives off camera, we described the points that we wanted to make. It went well.

Then it was on to the elementary school where the boy had been shot. What would we find? How could we help? We practiced looking calm and modeling self-control. Police and media were in the parking lot, and it was difficult to ge into the building, but we found the building to be calm and orderly.

The principal emphasized that most students had remained calm when they were told of the shooting, only a few students had been really upset, and those students were referred to the counselor. It was emphasized that the boy who had been shot was at the hospital and would be fine. He had been shot in the arm. The principal explained that she had been in a meeting at the central office when the shooting had occurred. She and the superintendent had immediately rushed to the school and had made several immediate decisions to establish control. Those decisions were the following:

1. All students were to be told in age-appropriate terms what had happened.
2. All schools in our district and area were to be alerted about the gunman.
3. Parent telephone calls and visits would be handled as well as possible. All doors were locked, and a policeman would stand at the front door. All visitors were escorted upstairs to the administrative area.
4. Students were kept inside all day and were kept away from windows.
5. Media representatives were not allowed inside the school or on school grounds. The police assisted with this task.
6. A note was sent home to each parent describing the incident and assuring parents that every effort was being made to ensure safety.
7. The loading of school buses was supervised by police at every school in the district.

Several of the policies mentioned above were part of an attempt to dispel rumors. Schools can always deal with the facts but cannot deal effectively with rumors. The physical layout of the school actually helped to allay the concerns of the many parents who came to school. The school is an open-concept campus with an administrative balcony that overlooks the entire school. Parents could locate their child's reading or math group and see that he or she was safe and that school was going on with normal activities.

It was very comforting after the incident to have police on all campuses and following buses home. We were told that at the alternative school, when students had seen three police cars in the parking lot, they had thought a drug bust was in progress. On such a dark day, even that little bit of humor was appreciated.

The next morning before school the superintendent and psychological services personnel spoke to the faculty of the elementary school. The faculty seemed very sad and appeared not to have slept well. We emphasized that the school children had probably slept better than they had. Plans were made for school that day.

The gunman turned himself in to police later that same day. The only statement that he ever made was that he had been angry at the world and had decided to take it out on children.

The boy who had been shot spent several days in the hospital. He received a get-well call from the President. He recovered completely both physically and psychologically.

For psychological services, however, the incident highlighted four points:

1. Communication channels needed to be clarified.
2. Alternative communication systems besides the telephone needed to be located.
3. Procedures to deal with the media and parents needed to be developed.
4. Crisis intervention needed to be added to the job description of personnel such as school psychologists.

What actually happened, however, was that we went back to business as usual in the school district. The consensus seemed to be that a terrible crisis had occurred but that nothing like this would ever happen again. As far as we are aware, the district did not develop new programs or procedures as a result of the incident.

Almost exactly 1 year later, as psychological services staff were enjoying a Friday lunch away from the office, our secretary rushed in to say, "There has been a shooting at the high school." A beautiful new high school in a nice neighborhood had been the scene of a shooting. We learned that the assistant principal had been shot in the cafeteria in front of over 600 staff and students. Reactions swung from shock to anger because the assistant principal was someone well known and liked.

This time we were wanted immediately to help out. We were flooded with panic and anxiety. What did we know about helping people at the scene of a shooting?

The Life Flight helicopter and an ambulance were leaving the school grounds just as we arrived. There were also two local television helicopters in the parking lot. We entered the school and went to the cafeteria area. A number of policemen and school officials were in the cafeteria; however, there were no students. They had left school or were back in their classes. Everyone seemed to be walking around in cricles. The spot where the gunman had stood was pointed out, as was the spot where the assistant principal had fallen. A student also had been hit by a bullet that had ricocheted off the wall. Everyone seemed to be processing the events in an attempt to come to grips with the reality of the situation. After about 5 minutes, we realized that we needed to be thinking about the emotional aspects of the event that had just happened.

Students and faculty members must have been experiencing some major emotional recoil from the incident. Facts picked up in incidental reading came to mind: approximately 25% of those who experience a crisis never resolve it; children are at highest risk; and the sooner startled students can express their emotions, the better off they will be.

Media representatives roamed the building. They were attempting to obtain a copy of the school yearbook with a picture of the 16-year-old gunman. The young man had turned himself in to the principal and had been taken away by the police. The principal was very much in demand. Everyone wanted to talk with him: the superintendent, counselors, media personnel, police, teachers, administrators, and our public information director. The principal could not do everything and had to delegate duties to others. One of the psychologists approached him and indicated that we had some ideas to assist the students and faculty. The principal stated that he was too busy to talk. However, he suggested that we write the ideas down. We penciled some suggestions with the sense that we were being "brushed off." In the end, however, the principal followed every one of these recommendations:

1. Keep students where they were for the remaining two periods.
2. Announce to all concerned exactly what had happened and provide updates on the medical condition of the victims.
3. Students who were to be interviewed by the police should be accompanied by an adult.
4. Individual and group counseling should be available to students as needed.
5. Students would have to return to the cafeteria to recover books, belongings, etc., that had been left behind.
6. A faculty meeting needed to be held after school.
7. Plans had to be made for the next school day.

It took some time to understand exactly what had happened. Apparently a 16-year-old honors student had made numerous references to his friends about shooting one of the assistant principals. His motivation to do so remained unclear but seemed to involve providing a "favor" to the student body by taking care of someone who stood for discipline.

The gunman, G, had had no disciplinary record. His contact with this assistant principal had been very limited. He had been asked to cut his hair a few days before the shooting. G told at least three friends of his plan to kill the assistant principal. Those friends apparently did not take the threat seriously. They did not tell any adults about the threat. It is not difficult to learn from this unfortunate episode: Somehow we must convince students of the duty to warn, that suicidal and homicidal statements must be taken seriously, and that adults should be informed.

The morning of the shooting the gunman had announced that he had a .357 Magnum in his locker. He had repeated his statement about shooting the assistant principal. When the bell rang for lunch, G told his friend to go on to the cafeteria ahead of him. He indicated that he needed to go to his locker. G then got the gun, hid it in his book bag, and joined his friend in the cafeteria. He ate lunch and left the cafeteria with his friend.

They then started wandering in an unfinished part of the school and were told to return to the cafeteria. It was then that G put on sunglasses and black gloves. He pulled the pistol from his book bag and shot the assistant principal in the side. He fired a second shot across the room at another assistant principal. The second assistant principal ducked, and the bullet that ricocheted off the wall struck a student in the leg.

Students dove under tables and fled from every exit. Their response was very reasonable, although many of them later expressed remorse that they had behaved in what they subsequently viewed as a cowardly manner. Some students felt that they should have grabbed the gun and have prevented the shootings. A few students felt they should have somehow read G's mind and known what he was planning. Several students had prior knowledge of his plans, and they felt very guilty about what had happened.

Everyone evacuated the cafeteria quickly. G walked around the cafeteria with what students described as a crazed but happy look on his face. This visual memory of the shooting scene stayed with students for a long time. Meanwhile, the school security guard rushed into the cafeteria, and G pointed his gun at him but did not shoot him. The security guard did not have a gun and fell to the floor, thinking he would be shot. The gunman left the cafeteria and walked outside. He heard police sirens and decided to reenter the school. The principal of the school blocked the entrance and somehow convinced the gunman to turn over his weapon and surrender to authorities.

Students were allowed to return to the cafeteria after school to retrieve their personal possessions that had been left behind. Many students who had left the campus did not return that day. A number of students did not return for several days.

A faculty meeting was held immediately after school. Everyone heard the details of the shootings and got a medical update on the victims. The student who had been shot was in good condition, whereas the assistant principal remained in serious condition. Everyone prayed for the recovery of the assistant principal, and the prayer seemed to help, as did making plans for how to proceed on Monday.

The director of psychological services spoke to the faculty that afternoon and offered individual attention to anyone who wanted to stay after the meeting. Only one person stayed to talk privately, and her concern was for her own son, whom she felt had serious problems and was capable of violence. The vast majority of the staff seemed to be in a hurry to leave school, go home, and forget.

For most of the faculty, escape from the school did not bring the relief that they hoped. Many of them felt vulnerable and afraid: any one of them could have been the victim. A shooting at their school had violated their expectations, and their normal coping abilities failed. In each faculty member unique memories of crisis and loss were stirred. Such haunting memories caused all of them much anxiety. We wished faculty members had stayed after school to talk. The literature recommends immediate discussion of personal reactions and provision of support. In retrospect, it seemed that everyone at the school in some way had felt victimized.

It was decided that a psychologist would follow the schedule of the gunman and answer the students' questions and that extra counselors and psychologists should be at the school to counsel students. In hindsight, however, we believe that we should have provided more immediate assistance by opening the school to students and parents on Saturday to talk about the shooting. This thought did not occur to anyone in the immediate aftermath of the crisis. It is difficult to think clearly when a crisis has occurred.

Many points made by the National Institute of Mental Health became very clearly apparent. "Children are resilient" was an important one, and the students did bounce back and recover well. The point about working with parents turned out to be excellent: The staff helped children most by helping their parents. It also became clear how necessary it was to seek out those students needing assistance. In a school setting this meant being in the hallways and classrooms so that psychologists could locate the students in emotional duress who needed to talk.

On Monday morning G's schedule was followed, and questions that his classmates asked were answered. The students wanted to know why he had done what he did and what would happen to him, questions for which there were no immediate answers. The judicial procedures undertaken when a juvenile commits a serious crime were explained. The district attorney had announced intentions to have G certified to stand trial as an adult. Rumors had to be dispelled: that G had posted bail, was out of jail, and would be returning to school. A medical update was given to students that informed them that the assistant principal would survive but that he faced a long rehabilitation process.

Many counseling efforts were then implemented to assist the students. There were three basic tasks: (1) assist students who were in attendance during the crisis with their emotional reactions; (2) convince students who were afraid to return to school to do so; (3) assist the small group of students who were close to G, as some of his friends had prior knowledge of his plans and felt very remorseful.

It was clear that students and parents alike experienced a wide range of emotions following the crisis. Most students expressed sadness at what had happened. Teachers were most comfortable assisting students who were sad. The students who were in a state of shock or who laughed about the recent events were more difficult for teachers to handle, and they were referred to the counseling office.

One student stated repeatedly, "I don't care if he dies because I never liked him anyway." We initially thought the student was being defensive and perhaps didn't want to deal with past losses in her own life. This did not prove to be the case. Her attitude was, needless to say, very upsetting.

The students who had prior knowledge of G's plans felt very bad and felt that the incident could have been prevented. They reasoned that if they had told an adult, G's locker would have been searched and the lethal instrument removed. He had sworn them to secrecy, and they simply had not believed what G has told them could really happen. Many of these friends seemed to need private counseling and the comfort of being close to family support. One father returned from out of state to offer such support.

Media representatives conducted a number of interviews at the high school with administrators, psychologists, and counselors. The school was portrayed in a very favorable light and its personnel as truly caring individuals, dedicated to helping the students. One of the television stations did a segment on school violence. The segment contrasted the caring response of our district with another school district that had a teacher shot the previous week. The second system was portrayed as dong very little to assist students and having no plans to prevent such incidents in the future.

Counseling efforts continued for weeks and, in a few cases, months. Several incidents revived memories of the shooting in the minds of the faculty and students. These included those times when G was certified to stand trial as an adult, when the trial opened and concluded, and when the injured assistant principal returned to the school.

On the last day of school, several students staged a prank in the cafeteria. They dropped a cherry bomb firecracker from the balcony onto the floor in the cafeteria. Many students thought that it was a gunshot and evacuated the cafeteria. Many relived the earlier shooting. I am told that the assistant principal went out to the parking lot and asked the students to return to school, saying "If I can face this, you can also; lets go back in and have school."

The principal of the high school disciplined the perpetrators of the firecracker incident by having them begin the next year at the district's alternative school. The principal also made the decision that the school yearbook would not contain information about the shooting. It was felt that students should remember the year for other reasons, and this could best be accomplished by not mentioning the shooting in the yearbook. The principal also felt strongly that this incident could have been prevented and focused several school-wide projects on bringing students and faculty closer together. The principal remained hopeful that these projects would change the school climate so that if students learned that guns were on campus, they would recognize the potential danger and alert an adult.

Numerous school personnel wrote letters to representatives of the judicial system that requested that G not receive leniency in sentencing. School personnel also testified at his trial. The sentence that G received was 4 years, total. He was paroled after having served 1½ years. School personnel felt that his sentence had not been severe enough. It is interesting to note that the state of California has subsequently legislated harsher penalities for crimes committed at school. The assistant principal commented that he felt very supported by the school district. He felt that everyone had really tried to assist him and his family through his ordeal. This contrasts with the nonsupport and rejection that Feder (1989) described when analyzing similar returns. He was, however, unhappy with the judicial system. He did not like the way that he was treated when he testified, and he did not feel that 1½ years in prison was enough of a sentence for the student perpetrator.

The school system vowed that G would not attend our schools on his release from prison. If G had tried to enroll, legal recourse would have been sought. However, G did not try to reenroll. This seemed best for everyone concerned.

The shooting incident described was very traumatic for the entire school system. Everyone who was present at the campus remembers vividly exactly what his or her response was. It has taken a great deal of time and effort for everyone to recover. Today, 8 years later, it is hard to believe that these incidents really happened. Again we find ourselves tempted to be lulled into a false sense of security by the notion that violent incidents of this magnitude do not occur in our schools.

The Need for Advance Planning

It is difficult to function effectively during a crisis, and the more planning that has been done, the more effective the intervention will be. Teamwork is also essential. No one person can handle a crisis of the magnitude of the one in this example.

Students often believe that a potentially suicidal or homicidal individual will never follow through on his or her statements. This point is absolutely critical to reducing homicidal and suicidal behavior on the part of students. Our task is really twofold: (1) to convince students that something tragic could happen and (2) to ensure that students look to adults for help and do not try to solve the problem on their own.

We believe that schools must learn from every crisis incident and must address themselves to doing better the next time. Almost every school system has "skeletons in the closet"—crisis incidents that have occurred and that could have been handled better.

The thought that such violence or crisis couldn't possibly occur in a school is very common in the limited crisis literature that addresses the schools. Indeed, we hadn't planned to deal with such events, and we did not have trained crisis teams, but we did the best that we could.

These tragic events did motivate the Department of Psychological Services to approach the superintendent about forming crisis teams on every campus. Administrators historically have been reluctant to develop crisis plans. In a recent survey of Alabama schools, Stevens (1990) found only one in four with a written crisis plan and stressed that schools "should not be caught with their plans down!"

The administrators in our district were motivated to develop plans to prevent and manage crisis situations in the future, and this book is largely a result of having to face these crisis events and others. Our crisis intervention program is constantly evolving and, we hope, becoming more comprehensive.

6

In the Midst
of a Building Crisis
Without Prior Planning

Most school districts do not have formalized, comprehensive plans for managing major building crises or disasters. During a noncrisis period, the need is often relegated to a low priority, and the necessary energy and assets required to build a comprehensive crisis system are not delegated. Frequently, mental health professionals as well as other educational personnel are summoned at the least advantageous moment: at the actual time of the crisis. It is imperative that the school district mental health professionals be prepared to intervene efficiently and effectively at this most difficult time. Even without any sort of formal district-wide plan, a general knowledge of crisis stages and needs allows the intervener an understanding of what to expect together with general operating procedures. Such knowledge can go a long way during an actual crisis. This is what this section provides.

Once such intervention steps are seen as effective and credible in an emergency, it is hoped that the school psychologist will have more opportunity to advocate steps in the direction of prevention. Thus, the general requirement for skills is actually twofold: (1) to establish crisis management procedures that support effective coping/management behavior during extreme emotional states and that will help to return the system to normal functioning as quickly as possible; and (2) to introduce crisis prevention activities that will reduce the probability that the crisis will recur.

Throughout this book, and certainly throughout the crisis plan, a continual push must be maintained to look beyond just "surviving" the present crisis. We must be a proactive force to use each crisis experience as a learning experience. Not only do advance planning and training aid us in the smooth management of a crisis that takes us by surprise but many sorts of crises might be prevented altogether through primary and secondary preventive efforts. Whereas the present chapter focuses on managing the immediate crisis well, Chapter 7, "Establishing a District-Wide Crisis Intervention Program," maintains more of a focus on prevention.

The overarching process of intervening with a building crisis can be similar to crisis intervention with individuals. However, when an entire building is in turmoil, the sheer quantity of demands is overwhelming. What complicates the picture significantly is that the emotional contagion of the professionals, students, and parents as they contend with the crisis may constitute a crisis in itself. The unfolding of the actions and reactions that a building or community crisis is, however, to some extent predictable.

THE CRISIS CALL

By definition, the crisis call is usually unexpected. Immediate action is necessary. The element of surprise, however, conveys with it the inclination to take action without careful thought to some of the crucial elements of the situation. When the call does come in, it is important to learn as much as possible about the nature of a crisis before becoming involved (Zizzo, 1989). Do not forget, as in any other crisis, to be sure to gather information about the incident and to communicate with those around you.

ARRIVING AT THE SCENE

What can you expect when you arrive on the scene of an organizational crisis or disaster? Probably the most pronounced aspect at this time is the intense emotional upset or "disequilibrium" experienced by the system. The "system" in this case could include almost an entire school and a good portion of parents in the community, or it could be limited to one class, the teacher, and perhaps some administrative staff. In any case, the intensity of emotion that greets you will probably at first require some mental preparation of your own.

Secondly, a flood of demands emerges: teachers want guidance; students need support and comfort; parents want information; everyone wants to be sure he or she is safe.

Many staff members "at the scene" may not react realistically or logically to the problems at hand no matter what their training or background. As with individual dynamics, denial or disbelief is the most common immediate reaction. Of course, denying that something hideous has occurred in your school and your life may provide some brief emotional protection, but the process of denial does not lend itself to logical decision making or plans of immediate action. Furthermore, sooner or later there must be acknowledgment that a significant loss has occurred. Then, as in personal crises, staff members and students alike experience feelings of helplessness, inadequacy, and confusion. It is difficult for anyone to think logically in the face of strong emotions. Often unresolved prior issues and losses surface, and the victims are flooded with waves of emotion depending on each individual's own unique crisis history.

For this reason, it is often productive to summon outside professionals to help manage the situation. However, the presence of the "outside" crisis helper or team has the potential either to escalate or deescalate the situation. People in crisis frequently have commented regarding the helpfulness of simply a calm presence to support them. It is important to remember that your effect as a model at this time can be tremendous; you must appear calm, confident, and supportive.

Traditionally, four patterns have been documented among students (Klingman & Eli, 1981). These, in our experience, can be counted on if an incident has shocked a large portion of the student body. If a severe incident has occurred, the symptoms may continue for days afterward. These are:

1. The rate of absenteeism is high just after the incident. Students become upset and leave the building in an effort to seek safety.
2. Children appear restless; they wander about; some are edgy and jumpy. This pattern is one that must be immediately contained. When students cannot be located, the panic over the crisis incident can snowball.
3. Children seek the company of adults (or peers, if adolescents) with whom to talk. Even the older "rough and tough" students usually need to take time out and discuss the incident to help process it mentally and emotionally. Many students will request to go to the counselor's office.
4. Complaints arise of difficulty with concentration and of stomachaches and headaches. If given the opportunity, many students will request to go to the nurse's office or clinic.

WHAT HELP WILL BE NEEDED?

Before you depart for the "scene" of the crisis, a quick assessment should be made to determine whether you have adequate manpower at the building to manage needs. How many individuals in addition to you will be required? It is far better to send more crisis helpers than are eventually needed than too few. However, your ability to do so will again necessitate that you know as much as possible about the situation before arriving at the scene. Again, we stress the importance of succinctly gleaning as much of this crucial information from your initial telephone contact as possible. How much support will be required to support the counselor and the nurse? What will the building policy be on allowing students to leave their regular classes? Should teachers be instructed to talk with students regarding the incident in class? How will teachers get word regarding the facts and how to discuss them with the students?

Our aim at this point is to manage the immediate crisis and support the school or even the district to return quickly to some form of "normal" functioning.

CONSULTATION WITH ADMINISTRATION

It is necessary to remember that the overall role you are in is that of a consultant. Basic principles of consultations still apply. It is important to (1) demonstrate interest and involvement in the situation, (2) invite and encourage participation, showing consideration for the other's feelings, and (3) maintain and demonstrate respect for the skills and professionalism of the school personnel.

Administrators may be looking for direction regarding management of the crisis. Most are uncertain about what to do; we feel this is why the most common response from most administrators is to ignore crises when possible. To maintain a consultative role, a five-step model outlined in Table 6.1 has effectively guided crisis intervention efforts in multiple mental health settings, including schools (Leviton & Greenstone, 1989; Greenstone & Leviton, 1982). It is presented in Table 6.1 as a step-by-step guide to decision making in the middle of bedlam.

Immediacy

This step refers to the significance of intervening as quickly as possible. This usually means you must be available, get to the building quickly, and work with the person in charge in that building or classroom. This person must make decisions and take action to restore normal function-

TABLE 6.1. Model for the Consultative Role

Immediacy	Intervene as quickly as possible
Control	Get control of the overall situation
Assessment	Complete a quick, accurate, "on the spot" evaluation of the situation
Disposition	Be sure that no one leaves without appropriate communication and information
Referral and follow-up	Anticipate future difficulties and plan how to allot resources for them

ing to the school or classroom immediately. Frequently this key individual does feel he or she knows what should be done but is waiting for support from another professional in making these decisions.

Control

The second and most critical step is establishing control of the total situation, even if it is artificial or unusual. A familiar voice that calmly instructs staff and students as to what to do goes a long way toward restoring faith that they are in good hands. This is crucial when emotions are running high and there may be mass confusion. The individual in charge should not attempt to explain what occurred or why at this point. What people need are concrete directions about what to do.

1. Contain the precipitating event. Should the police be called? Yes, if it is necessary to apprehend any ongoing violence. Remember, it is not the role of any crisis team member to take on responsibilities of the police. If a student or adult has violated the law, police should be called. If this is an individual, he or she should be physically apprehended or contained. If a portion of the building is involved, it should be isolated and students and faculty removed. Some districts may have security personnel who should also be contacted.

2. Get students and teachers to reasonable locations where they are physically and psychologically safe. They should be told approximately how long to remain there or when they will be given further information. If, for example, a serious knife fight has occurred in the cafeteria, it might be necessary for students to return to the fourth-period class and remain there for 30 minutes. At times "freezing" the schedule for a fixed period of time may be necessary if hallways or the building yards are in turmoil. Often students and school personnel may have scattered

throughout the building or outside. Students who may have left an assigned room or the building for any reason should be asked to return. Removing a class of individuals from a violent student may require temporary quarters for the duration of the crisis.

3. Should medical help be summoned? Yes, if there has been even questionable or minor injury.

4. Assign someone to keep a log of what is known to have happened and each step the crisis coordinator makes (e.g., police contacted at x time and arrived at x time, spent 2 hours inspecting the building).

Assessment

Once control has been established, one can afford a more careful assessment of the situation. An on-the-spot evaluation must be done. It must be quick, accurate, and must cover as many areas as possible to give total assessment of the state of affairs. Basic "who, what, where, and when" answers must be assembled in order to determine what will next be needed.

During what may be a brief interim in disorder, the individual in charge should consider what his or her needs may be for the remainder of the day. Depending on the nature and magnitude of the crisis, the following are all possibilities:

1. Contact should be made immediately with the central administration of the school district. Information should be provided as far as is possible. Sometimes this will need to occur via messenger or computer, since telephone lines are often jammed.

2. Are there any unmet medical needs? Students with minor physical abrasions, etc., may need attention.

3. Is everyone accounted for? In some circumstances students may have left the building and not returned. If possible, attendance should be taken and quickly processed. If individuals are missing, their parents should be contacted.

4. Are there any students experiencing such severe psychological upset that they will need to be removed from class and attended to? Where and with whom will they go? Such contacts might include any relatives or close friends of injured parties. Even if there are no available resources for attending to these individuals, it may be productive to remove them to a temporary supportive, private atmosphere.

5. What will be told to the parents and community? What information will be given over the telephone? How will you disseminate information to parents and the community?

6. What will be told to the media, and who will do it? If reporters come to the campus, where will you ask them to stay?

7. Someone will probably need to stay in contact with the police department, stay with them in the building to answer questions, gather information, etc.

8. What will students need to know about the incident before leaving school that day? How will this information be imparted to them (e.g., by their classroom teachers, over the loudspeaker, through some form of written information)?

9. What information or preparation will teachers need before leaving school that day. Stress felt by teachers is often relieved by simply having basic questions about what happened answered instead of permitting them to wonder all night about it. A simple "thank you" for their efforts and tolerance replaces feelings of confusion with pride at a job well done. Teachers frequently also need to have a simple, concrete plan of action for the following day.

10. When should the group of individuals working on these tasks next meet to discuss progress, steps to be taken, etc.? In almost every case, this group of individuals should meet prior to the close of the day.

Disposition

When this analysis is complete and appropriate steps have been taken, students, parents, and teachers will be ready to leave for the day under the best possible circumstances. The message that is important for all to leave with is, "We have had a serious problem today, and we have managed it well and are prepared for tomorrow" or "the school is under control, and should something like this ever happen again, it will not be pleasant, but we know we can again manage it competently."

Teachers and students should be praised for their part in managing the crisis. They should leave without many questions regarding the "what, where, and when" aspects of the incident without compromising confidentiality. Most importantly, they should leave with the feeling that the school is under control and safe to return to the following day.

The administrator or person in charge has also been through a harrowing day. Even the most independent of individuals responds to encouragement and support. Before the day is over a "processing" or "debriefing" period including all of the individuals who participated in managing the crisis is almost mandatory. It is frequently at this point, when the crisis is over and the immediate responsibilities and pressures have been alleviated, that anxiety is expressed through anger, slap-happy laughter, or sometimes tears. This is a natural and necessary part of the process.

Referral and Follow-Up

Referral and follow-up first must be considered regarding the immediate crisis. Many of the areas cited under assessment above should be considered for follow-up. The day after the crisis occurs carries with it the potential to be as hectic as the crisis day if various possibilities are not considered and prepared for. The following points should be considered:

1. Might there be an onslaught of parent contacts or visits? If so, where will they go, and who will be available to speak with them? Should a formal, evening parent meeting be scheduled inorder to answer questions, address concerns, and generally "debrief"?

2. Might there be numbers of students who are emotionally upset or who may become so throughout the day? If so, who will attend to them? Where will they go? Will you need to be concerned with separating those who are sincerely upset from the manipulators?

3. Would it be appropriate or feasible to structure regular group counseling meetings for students? Who will be in charge of this project?

4. Will it be necessary to have another staff meeting to answer questions, address concerns, or "debrief" during the day?

There is also a second frontier of referral and follow-up. This aspect relates to the willingness of the school, school district, or organization to prepare in advance for future crises. Shortly after a crisis occurs is a productive time to discuss these possibilities with administration or staff of a district or building. The memory of the incident and disruption is still clear in everyone's mind, and once involved with a crisis, the shock and potential complexities are clearer.

"Things we might have thought of and didn't"; "things we might have ready for next time"; "we were really lucky that event *x* didn't happen to complicate the situation further," are all very natural conversations that informally occur and assist in preparation for another crisis. It is a short step from there to adopting a building or district policy to formalize a plan for crisis.

CONSULTATION WITH TEACHING STAFF

Teachers usually need to meet before leaving that day. They should be told exactly what is known about the incident in order to dispel rumors. They should be supported and praised for their present efforts, strength in managing a difficult situation, etc., and be given a chance to "blow off steam" about the events of the day. They should also leave prepared with a plan of action for the following day.

Basic information should be given to the teaching staff to sharpen their awareness of the crisis/stress syndrome and give them direction in selecting classroom activities. Some basic helpful advice includes:

1. Acknowledge with the class the observable reality, give students information, talk about thoughts, feelings.

2. Provide opportunities to vent feelings.

3. Help students clarify the distinction between facts and comments, between news and rumors. (Suggestions for classroom activities to accomplish this are listed in Appendix A.)

4. Teachers need to know what to expect for reactions in their students. They should receive some direction regarding how to discriminate which students should be sent to the counselor's office and a rough estimate of the numbers of students that the office can accommodate (given personnel restrictions).

5. Teachers need to get the incident worked out for themselves so that they can be calm and reassuring to pupils. Any ventilation or emotional releases among staff should occur in the teachers' lounge after school hours and far out of earshot of the students.

6. Watch for stress reactions among teachers and "burnout" if the crisis is ongoing.

7. If teachers appear to have many questions or apprehensions about the situation, it helps to have a "roving consultant" available to answer, comfort, provide support, and encourage.

8. It may be helpful to offer group meetings with the teaching staff at noon and again after school the day following the incident.

A number of ready-made handouts for teaching staff are provided in Appendix A under the teacher liaison function.

Services to Parents

Usually a meeting with parents needs to be scheduled as soon as is practically possible following the incident. It may be necessary to continue to meet with parents for several weeks until the crisis has passed. Parents also should be told complete information regarding what is known about the incident. They will also need to know what to expect in terms of crisis reactions in their children and themselves. Handouts in Appendix A of this book may be used as a framework for information provided or to be dispensed to parents, even through the mail, if occasion demands.

Services to Students

Students may need brief crisis counseling either individually or in groups (see Chapter 2 for techniques). Teachers should be given guidelines for how and when to allow students to leave class for counseling, and extra support people will probably need to be on hand to help with the added duties.

What we have established in this chapter is a practical, quick plan for providing services in a crisis without preparation. However, with advance planning, a much more comprehensive and professional management can occur. Sometimes things have to get worse before they get better. As individual people, we know only too well that we frequently don't react to a problem until it becomes a crisis. As a society, we are no different. In many ways crisis intervention in the schools requires a system readiness to manage a variety of crises and ultimately to prevent them.

Frequently, the district readiness will peak just following a shocking crisis. Perhaps it is this aspect of school crises that offers the opportunity so frequently touted as part and parcel of crisis events. At any rate, the what and why of a larger, more-thought-out program is presented in the following chapter.

7

Establishing a District-Wide Crisis Prevention and Management Plan

Our profession generally has not prepared us to be proactive in establishing and organizing crisis intervention activities in the schools (Smead, 1985). School personnel, including school psychologists, are infinitely more amenable to primary or secondary activities once they have found themselves face to face with the tertiary prevention problems of managing a crisis. In reality, therefore, professionals frequently are faced with the somewhat illogical approach of beginning to intervene at the tertiary level of crisis management, and only later do they focus on primary and secondary prevention activities.

Of course even under the best of circumstances not all crises can be avoided. What's more, for those that can be avoided, as soon as we learn how to avoid them, new ones will take their place. This almost ensures that primary prevention, even in the theoretical ideal, should not be our sole aim. Secondary and tertiary prevention will always be necessary in the face of unpredictable natural disasters, bizarre violent acts, etc.

PRIMARY AND SECONDARY PREVENTION: GETTING AHEAD OF THE GAME

When all of the possibilities of crisis management and prevention are considered together, a task of much larger proportion emerges. It suggests that necessary areas of preparation, intervention, and research are not limited to the potential kinds of crises that might occur within a school environment. In fact, we must focus attention on these: (1) how to manage each particular crisis if it occurs completely without warning (tertiary prevention); (2) how to manage each particular crisis if it occurs with some brief warning; and (3) how to completely prevent the occurrence of a crisis when possible.

Conceived in this manner, the proposed task is clearly quite massive. This is why throughout crisis intervention literature the issues of teams of individuals and interdisciplinary cooperation are necessarily points of emphasis. Although it is certainly logical that mental health professionals would be key members of many crisis intervention activities, nobody can be a hero when comprehensively preventing or intervening with crises. Teamwork is the key if we are truly to promote the good of all.

GETTING ADMINISTRATIVE SUPPORT

To actually train and maintain a fully functional crisis team is a significant commitment of district resources and time. Administrators need to understand thoroughly the number of individuals, hours of training (both initially and on an ongoing basis), and ongoing time commitment that will be necessary to maintain a fully operational team.

Further, if crisis teams are to be available at each building, it will be necessary to enforce the responsibility and ensure that each building principal is invested in the effort.

Overcoming administrative reluctance to develop crisis plans and getting the support from a superintendent determine whether or not school systems are prepared for the inevitable crises that will occur. Our experience has been that all schools have had crisis situations, and that many school personnel wish they had somehow prevented the crisis from occurring or done something differently to better manage it. The following quote from Carden, the principal of an Alabama school where a gunman held hostages for 12 hours, illustrates administrative reluctance: "School officials are reluctant to face this. It's like a will—people are afraid to write one because they think they will die if they do!" (quoted by Jennings, 1989, p. 27).

McIntyre and Reid (1989) outlined several general obstacles to crisis planning in the schools:

- Myths and fears that taking proactive action makes the crisis worse.
- Territorial issues and conflicts as to whose job it is, both between school personnel themselves and between the school and community agencies.

- Lack of resources and not enough time.
- Few if any curriculum units for students emphasizing safety and problem solving.

Administrators have not been trained in crisis intervention. They are not prepared for the varied and complex crisis situations that occur in the schools.

Crisis situations represent a tremendous challenge for school administrators. It is essential that everyone in the school system work together to prevent and manage crisis situations. It is also necessary to coordinate school efforts with those in the community. Faced with such a complex task and a strong denial that it could happen to them, most school systems do not develop crisis plans.

We have consulted with numerous school personnel in positions such as counselor, nurse, or psychologist who were frustrated by what they perceived as a lack of support for their crisis intervention efforts. Our advice to them was to be persistent and aggressive. Plans need to be drawn up and submitted to the superintendent. We have provided 1- or 2-day in-services to numerous school districts on crisis intervention. The purpose of such in-services is not only to provide information but to motivate those in attendance that they can do something. Many districts have developed plans and taken action following the in-service. A few have not and have requested a second in-service. Those that did not take action shared a common denominator: the superintendent was too busy to attend the in-service. Leadership and support of crisis intervention from the superintendent are essential. We were very assertive in requesting that our superintendent appoint a committee to work on crisis intervention. We wanted to be on it, of course, but we were surprised when he directed the Department of Psychological Services to develop the plan for the district. We were very aware of territorial and political issues and solicited input from other departments and especially from building principals. The involvement of the abovementioned personnel was very helpful. Some of the pitfalls that we faced, which were discussed in Poland and Pitcher (1990), were the following:

- Principals attended the in-service on crisis intervention but initially did not form their building crisis team.
- After forming their crisis team, they held no further planning meetings on the campuses.
- No efforts were directed at how to prevent a crisis from occurring.
- No plans addressed how the building plans were coordinated with the transportation department.

- Crisis intervention simply was not viewed as an ongoing part of conducting school.

CRISIS DRILLS: MAKING CRISIS PLANS MEANINGFUL

Each of our schools has a crisis team. We had trained all their team members, but something was bothering us. No one seemed to be taking this as seriously as we felt they should. The important crisis planning had to be going on at the campus level—but was their planning being done? Would the principal remember to replace a crisis team member should he or she retire or transfer? Our crisis plan looked good on paper, but was it just something gathering dust on a shelf? We shared these concerns with our superintendent and deputy superintendent.

"Drills, that is what we need," suggested the deputy superintendent. He recounted an experience that he had in which an assistant principal had staggered into his office with what appeared to be blood on his shirt. It was in fact ketchup and was part of a class exercise on legal issues. He suggested that the psychology department could set up some crisis drills and that drama students could act out crisis situations to see how the schools responded. He commented that our schools were competitive, and that the psychology department could grade their crisis intervention efforts. We were concerned about the directness of this approach and did not want to give the schools a grade. We stated that we had worked for years to develop rapport with the principals and did not want to be in a position of assigning them a grade. His idea was a good one, but we needed to set it up so that it would not be too threatening. The purpose of the drill should be to ensure readiness and to provide a learning experience.

Historically, schools have had fire drills but no other types of drills. It is clear that many other types of crises occur besides fires. We suggested a paper-and-pencil activity to start with. A compromise was reached, and it was decided to conduct crisis drills. The principals were told the following:

1. Several surprise crisis drills would be conducted next month.
2. Central office staff would be on hand to role play the crisis.
3. The emphasis would be on a team response and on evidence of prior planning, and principals would receive both verbal and written feedback on their teams' response.
4. The drills would be videotaped to show at the next principals' meeting.

It was not difficult to write scenarios for the crisis drills. We simply looked through newspaper clippings of crisis events. The crisis scenarios for the first two crisis drills are provided in Appendix H.

The response of both the elementary and secondary schools were very thorough and did demonstrate much prior planning. The location of both hypothetical crises was by design outside of the school to minimize disruption. A number of surprise drills were conducted over the course of the next 2 school years. Scenarios dealt with such incidents as teacher heart failure, a near-drowning, and an automobile accident. The crisis visitation team had a sign made up that said, "Crisis Drill in Progress." We also learned to travel together in a van to avoid "tipping the school off." Principals often asked us when their campus would be visited. Our response was that the deputy superintendent decided which school we would visit.

Surprise Central Office Drill

The psychology department received a call from one of the principals who had been visited by the crisis visitation team. The principal felt that the central office had not been practicing what its members had been preaching and had not taken steps to prepare for a crisis at the central office itself. How would we like to participate in a surprise drill at the central office? We thought about our job security a moment and then agreed. The principal had come up with the rather ingenious scenario detailed below.

Incident

What appears to be an irate taxpayer has, after heated discussion in the tax office, kidnaped the tax assessor. As they exit the building, another employee is brushed aside while entering the building. She suffers an injury and collapses inside the front door.

A reporter from the *Monthly Moon* newspaper has stopped by and is in the parking lot, listening to an angry Hispanic woman whose car has been blocked in by two men in a maroon pickup truck.

From her view at the door, the employee who had been knocked down sees the kidnapper take the tax assessor to a maroon pickup. The last thing she heard him say as they left the building was, "Well, if you can't do anything about my taxes, maybe they'll let me talk to the superintendent."

Finally, the district security officer who is driving by has pulled into the parking lot to see what's causing the commotion.

Task

Please respond to this incident following the district crisis intervention procedures. District personnel are on the scene to role play and ask questions. This is a *practice drill,* and district personnel should be alerted, therefore, that it is *not necessary* to notify agencies outside the district.

Result

This surpise drill caught the central office completely unprepared. The deputy superintendent was out to lunch, and the superintendent was in a meeting; everyone was uncertain what to do. After a long delay, an employee who spoke Spanish was located, and the superintendent did come out to speak to the irate taxpayer. A good laugh was had by all who participated in the crisis. That afternoon, at the principals' meeting, it was announced that the first building had failed the crisis drill. The central office had been found unprepared, but it was recognized that a crisis could occur there, and steps would be taken to prepare for a potential crisis in the future.

The crisis drills heightened everyone's awareness of crisis intervention. The crisis intervention program came alive, and school personnel started thinking and planning. It has been very exciting to see school personnel come up with ideas and share them throughout the district. A few of the ideas that we would not have thought of were the following:

- Creating a crisis box with needed supplies in case a school has to be evacuated.
- Locating shelter in nearby businesses and houses of worship for students and staff who evacuate a school.
- Locating parents who live near the school and who are at home and can assist in a crisis.
- Establishing emergency medical teams in every building to assist medical liaison and teaching CPR and first aid courses on every campus.
- Utilizing the district computer system to communicate between buildings.
- Providing every principal with a red phone that ensures an outside line at all times.
- Developing a tip sheet for all employees to assist them in a crisis.

The crisis intervention program in the district has evolved and continues to evolve. Since their origination, the crisis drills have also evolved. The principals asked that they be allowed either to conduct their own crisis drill or to write up how they actually had handled a crisis.

The obvious advantage would be that crisis drills would take place in all 45 buildings rather than in the four or five that the crisis visitation team would visit each year. With some reservations, we decided to follow the recommendation of the principals. The principals would send a summary of their drill or their actual crisis to the Psychology Department for feedback. The department would record all summaries and ensure that every building documented its handling of a drill or an actual crisis each school year. The principals also asked for a crisis checklist to be developed to guide their actions. It appears in Table 7.1.

This procedure has been followed for 2 years with 100% compliance, but it has been necessary to remind principals. A concern has been that some of the documentation has not demonstrated a team response. A sample of the response that we are looking for appears in Appendix E.

TABLE 7.1. Crisis Intervention Checklist

1. Crisis coordinator (principal) becomes aware of crisis and notifies crisis liaisons.
2. Crisis coordinator clarifies duties of various liaisons and supervises crisis intervention activities.
3. Crisis coordinator or designee notifies superintendent of crisis.
4. Crisis coordinator interacts with media representatives as needed.
5. Crisis coordinator or designee notifies public information director of crisis.
6. Law enforcement liaison notifies security director and appropriate law enforcement personnel and coordinates their activities.
7. Medical liaison provides needed medical assistance.
8. Student liaison direct activities to ensure safety and emotional well-being of the student body.
9. Campus liaison communicates specifics of the crisis to the faculty and gives the faculty guidance on how they can assist in crisis management.
10. Counseling service or psychological liaison provides needed emotional support to affected students, family, friends, faculty, etc., as neeeded.
11. Parent liaison communicates to concerned parents verbally and/or in writing.
12. Teacher liaison provides assistance to classroom teachers during the crisis.
13. The crisis coordinator holds a faculty meeting to discuss the crisis after the students have gone home.
14. The crisis coordinator holds a debriefing meeting with the crisis team. This meeting processes the crisis event and clarifies follow-up activities for the team.
15. The crisis coordinator updates the superintendent and public information director on the resolution of the crisis.
16. The crisis coordinator discusses with the crisis team ways to prevent further crisis situations of this type.

Numerous actual crisis events have occurred, and they have been examined in terms of what could have been done to prevent the crisis or to have managed it better. Hypothetical crisis situations have dealt with natural disasters, sniper attacks, chemical explosions, and intruders in the school. Examples of such crises appear in Appendix E. The psychology department has assisted in setting up many hypothetical drills. An example of such a drill is described in a note home to parents that appears at Table 7.2

Crisis drills need to become a regular part of conducting school. Administrators need not fear that the public will criticize them for conducting such drills. We have not had one complaint from anyone's parents, staff, or students about our crisis drills. Crisis drills can save lives. This point was emphasized by Patricia Busher, the principal of Cleveland Elementary School in Stockton, California, where five children were killed and 29 others were wounded by a sniper on January 17, 1989. Busher stressed that previous drills had improved the children's response to the directives of adults and saved lives.

We encourage all schools to utilize crisis drills to prepare for crisis events.

WHY CRISIS TEAMS?

One major reason crises, especially those that impact at the entire school level or at community levels, can potentially cause such mayhem is the overwhelming need to attend immediately to many, many demands that

TABLE 7.2. Parental Notification of Crisis Drill

TO: Parents
FROM: The Principal
RE: Crisis Drills

It is our responsibility to have children prepared for any type of emergency. We have two fire drills per month and an occasional weather drill.

The Cy-Fair District recognizes that there are other types of emergencies that can occur in our society today. We must prepare students for these situations also. Therefore, today we had a drill pretending that an angry stranger entered the building and confronted our school psychologist. The drill gave us the opportunity to practice removing children from a potentially dangerous situation. The students responded very well.

The drill also reinforced the importance of having all visitors sign in and obtain a visitor's pass before entering the instructional area! Please cooperate with us in helping to ensure the safety of our children. Please call if you have any questions regarding today's drill.

---

are not part of our normal day-to-day routine. All this is occurring while the individual, himself, is still reeling from the emotional blast.

The idea behind the team approach is that no one person can do everything. Our administrators have emphasized that they could not be in four or five places at once, and, or course, without plans, which is exactly what they are being asked to do. First, it is not realistic that anyone should be expected to function at his or her best under these circumstances and to make wise decisions in the multitude of areas that will require attention. Second, so many matters typically require attention that it is physically impossible for any one individual to attend to them in a timely fashion. Usually it is this aspect of a crisis that we are most naive about. It has only been through experience that the requirements we have to enable us to handle a crisis have become apparent. We have mentioned these areas throughout the book. They are listed in summary below:

- Campus coordination, direction, communication with superiors, and logging of event and actions.
- Attending to students' needs.
- Medical emergency plans.
- Contacts, interactions with police, law enforcement.
- Contacts with parents.
- Contacts with the media.
- Correspondence with staff.
- Counseling services.
- Communication with other city or state officials.

Each one of these need areas can become a specialty in itself. At the time of the crisis, a great many activities can be completed in each area to optimally manage the crisis. Further, when the immediate crisis is resolved, primary and secondary prevention activities would ideally be formulated in many of these areas. In those areas not conducive to preventive policies or education, a great deal of "home work" could prepare a designated individual for the next emergency.

Figure 7.1 illustrates the potential roles necessary for a crisis team. The roles are conceived of in terms of "liaisons" or coordinators for that particular subspeciality of activities.

Appendix A includes a listing of qualifications, tasks, and sample materials pertinent to each of these roles. Before actually designating individuals to perform these potential crisis duties, some other broad-based issues should be considered.

Community, Central, or Building Crisis Teams

One question that should be given some consideration is whether these teams should be formed at the community, district, or building level.

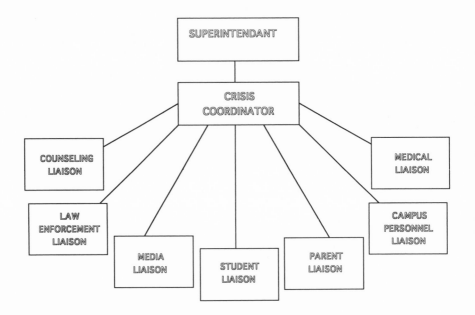

FIGURE 7.1. Possible elements and structure for a crisis intervention team.

Schools have three basic choices to develop crisis teams (Ruof & Harris, 1988):

- A *district team* involves personnel who only work for the school district.
- A *community team* involves school and nonschool personnel such as the police, fire department, medical, or mental health personnel.
- A *building team* is composed of only school personnel working in one building.

A second and somewhat related consideration is the expected frequency of events that will be labled "crises" or disasters. Most crisis team members cannot be expected to keep up with training and preparations when the incidence of crises is so low as to make the task appear fairly fruitless. In more rural areas, a community team might be a practical consideration. In such a case team coordinator might expand the size of his or her area to be sure that frequency keeps the individual alert and active to his or her role. In a large urban school located in a "high-risk" neighborhood, major building crises may occur with reasonable frequency to warrant a full crisis team within the building.

On advantage to an in-building crisis team is that everyone knows each other and the students. More day-to-day crisis planning is possible with a building team. A district-team approach involves some team members who work in the building affected by the crisis and others who are called from other locations. One district that used this latter approach had a very upset crisis team because the school the student who was killed attended did not call in the crisis team. We recommended that they add a representative from that school to the team in the future.

A community and district team is probably the most difficult to organize and maintain. One district had a very elaborate crisis proposal that outlined activities for many public agencies. We suggested that the school district clarify and organize its roles and get its plan implemented before making elaborate plans with public agencies over which it had no control. Schools need to look at their size and resources to lay out workable crisis plans. Districts such as the one in which we work should have building crisis teams. Medium-sized districts will need to use district personnel from more than one building. Small school districts need to locate personnel in their community or county who can serve on the crisis team.

A crisis plan should be laid out that is practical and clearly articulated. It need not be 250 pages. It should be simple enough for everyone to understand. Crisis intervention efforts need to be evolving and continually reviewed. No one will review a 250-page manual on a regular basis. A logical time to review and update crisis plans and discuss team member roles is after a crisis occurs. What can we do to prevent this from occurring again? How can we improve our response?

In any event, some of the liaison functions, almost by definition, must be carried out by professionals housed at each individual campus. These include:

- Coordination and direction of the building.
- Contacts with parents.
- Contacts with staff.
- Contact with individual in charge of counseling.

Other team members especially trained to interact with the media, police, and medical personnel might be dispatched from a central location. Probably the most thorough approach, however, would be to designate a crisis team at each building level and a second "backup" team at the overall district level. This method allows for a "teaming of the teams" with one professional in each area very knowledgeable about that particular campus (the building-team member) to work with a district-level individual who would in theory have more experience with various emergencies all over the district or county. The district- or county-team member could be called for consultation or hands-on help by the local, building-team member if deemed necessary.

Team Size

How many members should a crisis team have? Ruof and Harris (1988) suggest a minimum of one team member per 100 children. Poland and Pitcher (1990) discussed this question and recommended a team of four to eight members. More than eight is too many people to coordinate with, although some districts have teams of as many as 25 members. A team of two or three is not enough to delegate specific responsibilities. Further, if even one member becomes unavailable (e.g., sickness, absence), the team has suddenly become significantly diminished.

THE OVERALL ACTION PLAN

An overall action plan should consist of the following components:

1. The plan should be approved by the district, reviewed by the entire school staff, and reviewed by parent organizations. Input from these groups should be seriously considered prior to finalization of the plan.
2. At the time of a crisis the team leader arranges a meeting and notifies the central administration that the crisis team is meeting.
3. At the meeting all available information is shared with members of the team. Tasks are assigned, and a beginning plan is made.
4. Team members contact the crisis team leader as new information becomes available to them and routinely to report progress according to the plan.
5. During this period, the teacher liaison is quietly alerting the staff at that building to the crisis and providing them with all known information. A faculty meeting is arranged as soon as is possible to disseminate information an also to glean whatever relevant information can be assembled from the staff.
6. The team leader makes sure that he or his record keeper is making a record of the plan and also logging information as reported by the team members.
7. The media liaison should use the log information to begin to formulate a statement for the media that can be updated as the day and week continue. Guidelines for this statement are included in the section on media liaison below.

A crisis intervention checklist is provided in Table 7.1 to serve as a further conceptual and pragmatic guide for executing a crisis plan.

COMMUNICATION ISSUES

Schools undoubtedly need a better communication system than they presently have, according to Stevens (1989). One major issue that schools face is how to communicate effectively *within* school buildings and *between* school buildings. A second major issue that schools need to address is how to communicate effectively with parents. A third major problem for schools is how to handle the media and how to establish a cooperative relationship with the media that will not result in false information being transmitted or the school being portrayed in a bad light. Two old sayings illustrate these points:

1. What happened when the boarding house blew up? Roomers were flying everywhere.
2. The superintendent said to the new principal, "I am not going to hold you accountable for what you say to the media, *but for what they say you said!*"

Seven years ago our district only relied on telephones for communication, and the principal with an emergency was no more likely to get a phone line to make an outside call than the teacher in the lounge who wished to check to see if his car repairs were done. Today, the following communication equipment is in use:

1. Principals have a red phone that guarantees them an outside line.
2. Every building has a computer that can transmit and receive messages to and from all other school buildings.
3. Principals and assistant principals at secondary schools have two-way radios.

The National School Safety Center has additional communication suggestions for schools.

1. Modernize intercoms and make certain that portable buildings are reached by intercom.
2. Have portable phones available.
3. Utilize fax machines.
4. Develop an emergency communications kit.

It is also important that administrators have available bullhorns to enable them to speak loudly enough to disperse or direct groups of students. Playgrounds and parking lots should also be covered by the intercom system. School buses also should have two-way radios so that bus drivers can get assistance without depending on a passing motorist. Future technology will probably give administrators more tools to utilize in a crisis. Schools need modern equipment to cope with the variety and number of crises at school.

Our schools have also worked on communication within the building. Such communication typically involves a code word to summon members of the building-crisis team or to alert teachers to a particular danger. The code words are used primarily in the elementary schools where the administrators do not use two-way radios. The use of such codes needs to be practiced regularly to avoid the confusion involved in the scenario below.

> The secretary became very flustered at the many demands being made by the television reporter. She used the intercom to call for administrative help and unfortunately used the exact code that had been designated to indicate that the school was under sniper attack. Children were immediately evacuated from the playground, and blackboards were pushed in front of windows within seconds. The school was prepared for the sniper but not for an aggressive reporter.

What if you don't have an intercom system at all? Teachers need some way to communicate with the office. Teachers can not leave injured students and run for help. The buddy system and common sense would say that you alert the nearest teacher to assist you. But what if you are isolated, as in a portable building? We suggest the following communication system be worked out in advance using reliable students. The responsible student takes a card with the teacher's name on it directly to the office. A red card means a medical emergency; a blue card signifies an administrative emergency.

TRAINING CRISIS TEAM MEMBERS

Over the past 30 years, recognition of the importance of crisis intervention skills has increased significantly (Hoff & Miller, 1987). Volunteers, citizen's groups, and mental health professionals have come to recognize that neither piecemeal training nor academic degrees necessarily prepare or qualify them for doing crisis intervention. Recently the Surgeon

General's Workshop *Final Report* (1982) recommended that victimology and crisis intervention be included in the curricula and licensing examinations of all health and human service professionals.

Hoff has presented a list of "core" education necessary to basic effective functioning in crisis intervention. She divides these core training needs into three domains: knowledge, attitudes, and skills. They are listed in Appendix C (Reproduced with permission from Hoff & Miller, 1987).

Appendix A of this book includes possible suggestions for the functions of various team members. Although the true nature of possible crisis organization is elaborated in the next few pages of this book, even a cursory review underscores the tremendous potential involvement these crisis management and prevention techniques might entail.

Personal Characteristics, Reactions, and Limits of the Crisis Worker

When crisis occurs, teachers, counselors, administrators, and all staff need to be ready immediately to cope with their reactions and the reactions of their students. This need to deal with and manage student reactions comes at a time when staff members may themselves be experiencing rather extreme emotional reactions. The more individuals are educated regarding what reactions to expect and what reactions are normal, and certainly what, in a very concrete manner, is expected of them, the more effective they are likely to be in overriding their own emotional reaction and maintain a focus on constructive methods to cope.

The success of a crisis management team can depend heavily on the selection of the team members. These individuals will be asked to put a significant amount of time into the effort. The roles provide excitement and many rewards, but there is also considerable stress. The jobs should not be forced on individuals who are not motivated and interested.

In crisis intervention, as in any helping field, there are various personal needs that can potentially greatly interfere with one's ability to intervene effectively. If the crisis interventionist tends to function in any of the following ways, he or she will seriously undermine his or her own efforts and those of the team. It is important for those dealing with crises to be open and alert to avoid these tendencies. The most significant in our experience are listed below:

1. The need to be a hero.
2. The need to be in control.

3. Difficulty tolerating unhappiness or strong emotions in others.
4. Taking on too much responsibility for the organization.
5. Discomfort with consultation, indirect roles.
6. The need to have things go perfectly.

Understanding Each Job and the Importance of Teamwork

Teamwork is important in carrying out all educational and mental health work. In high-risk or high-pressure situations, at least two team members should be present for support (e.g., a highly charged, angry parent meeting where parents charge that school staff acted irresponsibly).

Teamwork is also vitally important in supporting other team members during crisis work. Strain is unavoidable when working with life-and-death matters on an ongoing basis and frequently under time pressure. If a student commits suicide, the crisis team member at his or her building may need support.

Each crisis team member needs to be sensitized to the importance of intervening and coordinating as a team. Everyone must understand that there are several courses of action that will work against the efforts of everyone else. One is certainly acting alone and/or failing to stay in touch with coordinators or other liaisons. Confusion is generated from this pattern, and individuals who continually lean in this direction are not productive crisis team members and would probably function more effectively in another role.

Overall obsessiveness is another potential adversary to establishing a well-functioning crisis plan. Becoming too academic and believing that it is necessary to understand every detail about crisis/disaster preparedness is one guise such obsessiveness might take. Another is making very complex plans or establishing very complex organizations. Generally there should be no more than eight individuals on the crisis team itself. Larger teams generally do not hold up well when individuals are in crisis. The plan must be simple, and the role of each crisis team member must be very clear, concrete, and easy to remember.

Another key that should not be overlooked is the need to provide considerable recognition and compliments to members of the crisis team. Letting go of such recognition promotes burnout. The chance to recognize everyone's involvement and successful management not only promotes a positive image to the community but keeps the team energetic.

IDENTIFICATION OF TEAM LIAISONS AND CLARIFICATION OF DUTIES

The crisis team might function on a district level or at a building level. Indeed, some team members might be district-wide in a small district, whereas others would be appointed on site in each building.

Team members should be selected on the basis of each member's expertise. This list will likely include administrators, school psychologists, counselors, and other staff members not responsible for classrooms. Each individual should be willing to contribute several hours preparing for his or her role *in advance.* Thus, each person must be relied on to complete the "homework" deemed appropriate to his or her building/district situation. Ideally these individuals should be available to stay after hours to plan for crises and also to complete the necessary activities in the face of a real crisis. Therefore, individuals who have children who must be picked up or another job will need to take these matters into consideration before becoming involved.

It is essential that there be a team leader who functions with authority. This individual is responsible for making important decisions regarding possible courses of action for all the team members. Without this decision-making authority, and authority over the individuals functioning on the teams, the ability of the team to act immediately can be hampered severely.

Written Procedures

Each crisis team member should develop written procedures and materials for his or her role. A backup person must be able to use this information to operate in her or his place if necessary.

Campus Liaison

The campus liaison directs and coordinates the activities of the crisis team and corresponds with those in positions of authority in the school district and the community. Each team member reports major events and progress regarding the crisis to the campus liaison.

One of the primary duties of this crisis team member is to maintain the log of events and actions taken as the crisis and postcrisis reactionary stages occur. This record becomes indispensable for developing press releases, reporting to district administration, and keeping track of what is occurring at a time when memories may not function at their best.

The campus liaison must also remain available to make decisions regarding concrete direction for possible courses of actions of the crisis team members, for example, "I think you should call the police immediately." For this reason, the individual filling this position should have some authority in the school—probably the principal or a designate.

Counseling/Student Liaison

The counseling/student liaison role is really twofold: (1) to provide consultative support to regular teachers, "emergency" teachers, and parents, and (2) to provide direct group counseling skills for the screened students most in need.

It is crucial, then, that the counseling/student liaison work closely with parent and teacher liaison team members to be sure all groups are receiving the proper information and support to soothe the children's emotional reactions in the most natural environment.

During and immediately following a disaster or building crisis, most students, especially those most directly involved with the incident, will experience a great deal of confusion and emotional turmoil. The initial line of support and counseling is in the most natural environment: first from parents and second from teachers. With appropriate, informed attention and support from these significant others, the vast majority of children adjust with time. The major shock generally passes within 1 to 6 weeks.

Thus, the consultative function of the counseling/student liaison, working with the parent liaison, is to provide the needed mental health to these groups of "front-line" consultees. A system must be developed to provide teachers and parents the information and support they need. Only more serious problems that cannot be managed in the classroom should be referred for further in-school or private counseling.

Role of the Family

Even when a more serious case has been properly referred for counseling, a basic principle in working with a child, even in disasters, is that there is likely to be a family problem. Parents may need increased support in the form of family therapy (possibly through community agencies if not available within the school system), conferences with the school psychologist, counselor, or other professional, or parent group meetings that can be organized through the district crisis plan (parent liaison).

A substantial minority of children experiencing a disaster will suffer short-term emotional problems. Parents need to be informed beforehand of the possible disaster-related responses they might see in their children. During the impact phase, children should be united with their families as soon as possible and will need parental support. During the weeks just following the disaster, parents should spend increased amounts of time with their children, offering a calming influence. The parents need to hold their own emotional reactions in check and discuss anxieties and fears with other adults well out of earshot of the children (Perry, et al., 1956). This can be extrapolated to other adults close to the child such as the teacher.

Just following a crisis or disaster, some populations of students might require special outreach attention. They include students directly exposed to the incident who are not attending school, students already known to be functioning with emotional handicaps, and students who have been known to have gone through an ongoing exposure to intense stress in the past (death, divorce of the parent) or who are for historical reasons considered at high psychological risk.

Based on various screenings, a subset of students may be invited to participate in time-limited support groups. These are students showing significant functional, emotional, or behavioral impairment directly related to the immediate crisis situation.

Reactions to crisis vary according to age and developmental level, of course. Parents, teachers, and support professionals should have a thorough understanding of what reactions are normal reactions to crisis and generally how to manage them. In Appendix A is an outline of the variations in emotional reactions to crises across various age groups (adapted from Lystad, 1985).

In summary, crisis workers need to keep in mind the importance of working with parents to help their children, and must seek out those who need their services. The first point is well illustrated by the analogy of the airplane flight attendant who tells the parents of small children to put the oxygen mask over their own faces first. Children's reactions to crises can best be summed up by the work "regression." It is important that parents undertand and respond to their child with patience and tolerance. This is difficult for parents to do because the crisis has affected them as well. The second point is that we must seek out those who need help. We cannot wait in an office for them to find us.

Medical Liaison

The building nurses in our district serve as medical liaisons. They are an extremely motivated group. Those in the medical field simply are more motivated to prepare for crisis situations. Nurses can organize emergency medical teams within a particular school or within the district. More specific examples of duties are provided in Appendix A.

Law Enforcement/Security Liaison

The link between law enforcement and the school might at first consideration appear to be pretty straightforward. However, complications arise quickly if the school has had little prior experience or relationship with the local police and with criminal activity within the schools. Several issues that are likely to arise are outlined below.

The question arises as to when to report an incident to the police. Traditionally, schools independently have taken on the responsibility of keeping students' behavior under control. Thus, as criminal activity within the schools has increased, administrators have often dealt with infractions as a violation of school rules. However, if we are to work in tandem with community efforts to curtail juvenile crime, identification of offenses that are criminal acts in addition to being school infractions is absolutely necessary. We must become sophisticated in discriminating between school misconduct and school crimes (National School Safety Center, 1988).

Another problem area concerns staff/community adverse reaction to police in "their" schools. However, if the school is aware that there are dangerous, unlawful activities within the building and does nothing to stop them, the school could be found liable (*Stoneking v. Bradford Area School District*, 1988) because of violations of students' rights to "liberty" under the 14th amendment. If school officials demonstrate "due diligence" in preventing crime on campus, they are protected from being found liable in the courts.

The U.S. Supreme Court has concluded that school officials do not have to conform to the same stringent standard required of law enforcement personnel in regard to search and seizure: a warrant or the standard of probable cause does not need to be met before searching a student. School officials must, however, have "reasonable grounds" to suspect that a search will result in evidence.

Media Liaison

It is alarming and somewhat puzzling that the media often pick up on a real or imagined crisis before many of the school personnel are aware of it. A spokesperson needs to be identified to work with the media. Strategies to deal with this are discussed both in the section on communication issues (above) and in Appendix A.

Administrative journals have had numerous articles that have encouraged preparation for dealing with the media. How should one respond to the media? What should the media be allowed or not allowed to do at school? Bark (1989) cited media consultants who emphasized the importance of being honest, but he also recognized that the interview is a two-way street. Elliot (1989) made the following suggestions for the schools:

1. Mobilize resources quickly.
2. Involve the superintendent.
3. Show concern to everybody involved.
4. Share information with everyone involved.

Elliot contrasted the minimal and delayed response of the Exxon Corporation following the Valdez oil spill with the prompt, comprehensive, and caring response that the Johnson & Johnson Corporation had following the 1982 Tylenol® deaths. The Exxon Corporation head took a week to respond and initially sent a very small crew to clean up the spill. The result was to create a negative public image for Exxon. Elliot recommends that schools follow the abovementioned principles to give the public a positive image of how the crisis is being handled. Our administrators have stressed acting quickly and letting everyone know that you care and are taking steps to help people recover. Our superintendent also goes to the scene of the crisis.

St. John (1986) stressed the importance of a school having a single spokesperson to talk with the media to avoid having contradictory statements made by school personnel. St. John suggested making contact with the media before a crisis occurs and suggested the following:

- Compile names and addresses of the media.
- Develop a fact sheet on the district or school.
- Identify space at school where the media can work.

St. John also stressed prompt verification when a crisis occurs and then taking initiative and communicating with the media. Key points recommended are:

- Maintain a uniform position.
- Provide clear, concise, and prepared messages.
- Log all incoming and outgoing calls and personal contacts.
- Provide refreshments, equipment, and reasonable assistance to media representatives.
- Don't tell reporters how to write their stories.
- Make news releases brief and accurate.
- Handle negative events in a positive way.
- Don't ask to review articles before they are printed.
- Compliment reporters who do a good job.
- Know what is public information.

Jay (1989) also advocates a cooperative approach with the media. Communication lines must be open both within the school and between the school and the media. If the school administrator doesn't release a statement, someone less creditable will talk for him or for her. Jay advocates letting media representatives know what you are doing and what you have done. Poland (1990a) described opening a meeting held to discuss the suicide of a student with the statement that the school district had first initiated prevention policies 7 years before. Jay also recommends avoiding the use of bureaucratic language when talking with the media and stresses letting people know that you care. Further information about how to interact with the media is provided in Appendix A. Our experiences have underscored the importance of developing a positive relationship with the media but also setting limits as to what they can and cannot do at school.

Parent Liaison

Parents need and demand a great deal of attention when a crisis occurs within the school environment or community. When the crisis occurs within the school environment, parents need precise information on exactly what happened, assurance that it is indeed safe for their child to ba at school, and assurance that the professionals have a plan to provide the children with the help they may need. In a community-based crisis or natural disaster, parents may need support from the school district to help them cope appropriately with their children's reactions and needs or their own. Under many community-based assistance programs for victims of disasters or emergencies, the schools are an instrumental part of providing health, mental health, and supplies to the community.

A system must be set up to take and respond to calls. Telephone calls from concerned parents typically begin to appear startlingly soon after the incident, even before the media begin to broadcast any information regarding the crisis. Questions such as "Should I come and get my child?" "Is what I hear true?" or even "Put my child on the phone" can be so frequent that they block outgoing calls. Another system will probably be necessary to manage parents who drive to school on their own initiative and wish to see their child or to take him or her home. Thus, the parent liaison may need to identify several individuals who will be able to handle these specific operations just subsequent to the crisis.

Parent Meetings and Groups

Keeping the parents informed regarding a school-based crisis is an important key in maintaining their support and trust. Just as with the media, parents should be informed of all confirmed information as it becomes available. Rumors and overreaction to misinformation are frequent problems with crisis intervention; all efforts to keep all those involved informed undercut this tendency.

The parent liaison must have a devised method to inform parents of the meeting. Preprinted letters to be taken home with children are often the most effective method. This means, however, that the letters must be reproducible with perhaps only a few hours' warning. Advance preparation of a "boilerplate" letter can save a good deal of time when everyone is under pressure.

The meeting usually consists of the parent liaison team member, the crisis team coordinator, a district administrator (principal or even superintendent, if not already included as part of the crisis team), and the counseling liaison. The purposes of these meetings are several: (1) basic available information can be provided to parents regarding what happened and exactly what the district plans are for management; (2) any questions that remain can be answered; (3) parents can be allowed some input regarding what they would like to see the district doing; and (4) parents may be counseled regarding what to expect from their children as well as the most constructive methods for managing any unusual behavior or emotions.

For many more severe crises, more than one parent meeting will be required. The first should be scheduled as soon after the crisis occurs as is possible. The second might be scheduled a few days later in the same week. This allows those parents who missed the first meeting to attend the second before too much time has elapsed. Second, since parents' (and their children's) anxiety levels will be highest just subsequent to the crisis, information may need to be repeated or expanded on as it becomes available, further assurances made, and updates given on how students and children are progressing.

Another function of the parent meeting involves the opportunity for parents to discuss and share with each other regarding the incident. Advice from other parents is often more acceptable than advice from the "experts" or administration.

Telephone Crisis Lines

A temporary telephone "crisis" line often helps when large numbers of parents have questions that cannot be addressed at, prior to, or after parent meetings. For some families, the privacy of the phone lines offers a more acceptable way of obtaining support and information. Radio and television stations generally are pleased to help publicize the availability of a crisis line as a public service. Advertising the line as available to parents "to obtain information and suggestions regarding their children's fears and worries" usually draws a good response.

Past experience with these lines suggests that most problems can be met with telephone information as long as those manning the phones are professionals or well-trained paraprofessionals (volunteers). Local mental health agencies and colleges or universities can be sources of help in this effort. Those working with such phone lines in community crises or disasters have indicated that "the majority of the calls involve bedtime fears, clinging, and other behaviors that seem to reflect separation anxiety" (Farberow & Gordon, 1981, p. 32). Follow-up to the callers is also a desirable feature, with the caller being instructed to call back to provide an update on how the suggestions worked.

Teacher Liaison

The teacher liaison provides the basis of communication and training for teachers in the building. It is crisis intervention philosophy that the educational system is responsible for the mental health of the pupils and the teachers' competence in managing their pupils' tension. In addition, the overall philosophy includes carrying out most intervention in the natural setting by persons most identified with this setting. Thus, the first and most effective attempt to work with child victims of crisis is through teachers or counselors rather than through special psychological therapy.

Probably the first and foremost need of teachers is for precise, objective information regarding the incident. If the incident occurred on campus, each teacher should be aware of the facts relating to the incident (as far as they are known) before leaving the building.

Ideally, teachers will be educated before an emergency regarding children's emotional reactions to crisis, classroom activities for children in crisis, and the role of the teacher in a disaster. Sample training objectives for teachers and other school professionals are included in Appendix D. Once a crisis or disaster does occur, this information will probably need to be reviewed (prepared handouts are recommended) together with involvement of teachers in a plan for the following day.

Usually the teacher's tasks include:

1. Acknowledge with class the observable reality by providing comprehensive information.
2. Engage pupils in discussions and activities about their thoughts and feelings, letting them vent feelings and express reactions and communicate honestly.

3. Control their own emotional reactions to the students (it should be stressed that children take their own cues from adult figures).
4. Consult with counseling liaison regarding unusual or extreme problems.
5. Encourage and reward students for attending school even though they might be anxious or frightened.

There may be a small number of teachers who have difficulty carrying out these tasks. Individuals must be free to conduct such activities in the class with the teacher present and observing. Frequently these teachers will try to conduct their classrooms with the "business as usual" approach with total ignorance of the event that has happened, avoiding open discussion, and over- or underreacting to student's emotional, behavioral expressions of anxiety or stress (Klingman & Eli, 1981).

At times of crisis, personnel are often too busy and can't conduct classroom activities and carry on routinely while affording enough personal time to comfort students. An avenue should be planned in advance to provide extra "pairs of hands" to help support the regular teachers. The source of this extra support will necessarily vary from school to school, but some possibilities include resource and reading enrichment teachers and aides (whose classes may need to be canceled temporarily) and substitute teachers who are "regular features" of the school.

These extra floating staff have, under some conditions, worked as an in-building crisis team that met to support the regular teachers and also worked with students coming into the counselors' offices on a walk-in basis.

Outreach Materials for Children, Teachers, and Parents

In preparation for acting as a community center during a disaster, a crisis that might occur in school or on the bus, schools should begin to build a handy supply of materials that could be quickly accessed at the time of crisis. This book contains many sample materials in the Appendices under the various headings of teacher, child, and parent liaisons. Also, Appendix F includes a number of ready-made manuals and materials that can easily be ordered, used for more personal crises among stduents and parents, and stored in case of a large-scale disaster.

Burnout

Professional burnout has been identified as a syndrome common with crisis workers. Frequently, tempted by the above needs, crisis workers can overextend themselves emotionally, physically, and mentally. As a result, 6 months later, the individual finds him- or herself exhausted and overspent. This phenomenon occurs frequently among staff working with children and their families (Farberow & Gordon, 1981).

Whether during a crisis or disaster or on an ongoing basis, it is important to provide crisis team members with as much support as possible. The crisis role is enervating. If the team is called from a central location, it is difficult from them to accomplish any paperwork since they may be interrupted at any moment. Those students and their families who are intervened with are not always happy and cooperative, and the demand for services often exceeds hours in the school day and limits of staff assigned to crisis tasks. Overwork and overcommitment appear to be the major culprits in the process. Symptoms are summarized in Table 7.3 (adapted from Faberow & Gordon, 1981).

There are several pointers involving crisis work that can prevent crisis team burnout. School personnel may want to avoid giving out their home phone numbers to crisis-prone or at-risk students. Giving them your number implies that you will be available at all times for all possible emergencies. This is simply unrealistic.

Similarly, school personnel should not attempt to provide services beyond the school day. Community services that are staffed for this purpose (e.g., crisis telephone, clinics) should be relied on for future

TABLE 7.3. Symptoms of Burnout

Cognitive
Slowed thinking, confusion, difficulty in making sound judgments and decisions, setting priorities, and evaluating own functioning

Physical
Physical exhaustion, sleep difficulties (inability to fall asleep or sleep through the night), stomach and digestive problems, disturbances in eating patterns (loss of appetite, compulsive eating), loss of energy, tremors, and various complaints regarding physical ailments (headaches, back/neckaches)

Behavioral
Restlessness, agitation, nervousness, inability to sit still, apathy, withdrawal, loss of ability to move, loss of ability for self-expression (talking or writing), slips of the tongue

Feelings and mood
Depression, irritability, anxiety, easily triggered and excessive rage, guilt, ready overexcitement

---

Source: Adapted from Faberow and Gordon (1981).

referrals. When communities are not offering these services, there is more of a problem. However, it is not realistic for school personnel to take on 24-hour responsibility for students in a crisis.

A number of district support mechanisms should also be in place. Compensatory time for extra hours put in should be provided, and individuals should be encouraged to use it immediately. Some sick leave should be allowed for "mental health" leave. The district might also consider possible rotation of staff so that "high-demand" roles get some relief.

There should also be a safe place for those involved to release tensions, anger, or frustration. A pattern of staff and crisis teams supporting each other should be nurtured.

Other, additional pointers are helpful to ward off stress in crisis-related tasks. These include limiting the length of the day, avoiding taking crisis work home after the day is over, spending off-work hours with friends and activities unrelated to crisis work, and giving oneself "treats" such as scheduling massages or those purely "fun" activities many are tempted to give up when working too hard (movies, shopping, taking time to enjoy a meal).

Staff should be aware of the burnout risk and burnout symptoms for crisis work and be looking for the very first signs. Staff should understand the importance of an overall healthy life style and its contribution to the ability to tolerate stress, including good nutritional eating habits, regular exercise, and avoiding the use of caffeine, nicotine, or alcohol.

At the first sign of stress, supervisors should discuss the symptoms privately with the staff. Stress can often be prevented by immediately cutting back on the amount of time and energy involved in the crisis activity. It may be necessary to order time off if the individual involved refuses to admit to stress or to leave the situation. The reason for this refusal is often guilt. Usually individuals are responsive to the interpretation that they will be of most help in the long run if they "take care of themselves" to stay effective. Reassurance that they will be welcomed back when ready to return and that they will be able to contribute much more at that time if they are able to take this break will usually be effective.

Transportation Procedures and Bus Safety

We realized in our own district that crisis teams had been formed and trained at each and every school building, but no attempt had been made to coordinate the building crisis teams with existing emergency procedures in the transportation department. This coordination is discussed in an article by Poland (1989b). The transportation department was very responsive to our efforts to coordinate with them. Appendix outlines some basic principles for the bus driver if a crisis occurs.

A very basic question is how safe are our school buses? An article in *USA Today* (1989, May 29) entitled, "Riders and Accidents on the U.S.A.'s School Buses," reported that 40 children are killed annually while boarding school buses and 10 children are killed while riding. Safety on school buses has been questioned since the May 14, 1988 bus crash in Kentucky that killed 27 people. Rota (1989) reports increased safety standards in some states with regard to emergency exits and fire-resistant exteriors. Also under consideration are the following:

1. Relocating gas tanks.
2. Phasing out older buses.
3. Installing more mirrors.

Berger (1989) also raised several other issues about bus safety and pointed out that buses built before 1977 did not have to meet federal safety requirements. These buses are referred to as prestandard, and estimates are that 22% of the nation's 350,000 buses fall into this category. Berger raised other safety issues and recommended the following:

1. Buses not be overcrowded.
2. Routine emergency drills for school buses.
3. A regular bus inspection program.
4. Two-way radios as standard equipment.
5. Screening and training for bus drivers.
6. More emergency exits and push-out windows and roof hatches to allow quicker escape.

One of the worst bus accidents ever involving school children occurred in Alton, Texas, on September 21, 1989 when a busload of Mission I.S.D. students were hit by a Dr. Pepper truck. The bus was knocked into a caliche pit, where 21 students drowned. This incident raises many questions about the number of emergency exits needed on school buses.

McEvoy (1988b) discussed the training needs of bus drivers and pointed out that few bus drivers have training in managing children, and they tend to view the task of driving and solving discipline problems as incompatible. McEvoy also emphasized that there is a high turnover rate with bus drivers that interferes with establishing a cooperative relationship between children and bus drivers. A number of suggestions were outlined by McEvoy:

1. Drivers need to compliment children for behaving well.
2. Policies should be enforced firmly while treating children with respect—a few clear simple rules are best.
3. Drivers should take responsibilities seriously.
4. Drivers should avoid arguing with children.
5. Drivers need training in communication skills and behavior management.
6. Drivers need the support of school administrators.

Horswell (1991) discussed 10 school districts' attempts to improve the behavior of students on the bus by mounting cameras inside the bus. The districts reported improved conduct on the buses as a result of the program even when the boxes that held the cameras were empty. Students could not tell whether their bus behavior was being filmed or not.

We asked our transportation supervisors if they had ever experienced a serious bus accident. The answer was yes; a busload of elementary school students was hit by a truck carrying a load of sand. No students were killed, but several students were seriously hurt. By coincidence a carload of our district nurses happened by on the way to a meeting and provided emergency medical aid. School personnel reported that everyone at the school wanted to leave school and go to the scene of the accident. Major communication difficulties were encountered first in locating the emergency phone numbers for each student and, second, in getting phone lines out from the school to call parents.

A second bus accident was also shared with us. This incident involved a minor accident where no one was injured, but the driver of the automobile that was struck by the bus was irate and engaged in a shouting match with the driver. Each student on the bus also had his or her own idea as to who was at fault. A very volatile situation was defused when an assistant principal came from the school and separated the irate motorist from the students and driver. This example illustrates how difficult a job it is that bus drivers have. They are all alone with many students and a great deal of responsibility. Thus, drivers need training in numerous areas.

The training program that was developed by the psychology department in our district consisted of training in three primary areas: those of behavior management, suicide prevention, and crisis intervention. The training began with a group of 30 bus drivers who had volunteered to participate. Psychologists reviewed materials on assertive discipline for bus drivers (e.g., Canter, 1987). Psychologists also rode school buses and interviewed drivers about their management concerns while driving. The behavior management training emphasized the importance of getting to know students and treating them with dignity. The following behavior principles were stressed:

1. Immediate consequences for misbehavior.
2. Consistency on the part of the driver.
3. Remaining calm and restating the expected behavior.
4. Frequent praise of appropriate behavior.
5. Providing rewards for appropriate behavior.
6. Clearly separating the misdeed from the personal worth of the student.
7. Ways to utilize eye contact.

The drivers were especially receptive to learning more about suicide prevention. Unfortunately, one of the district drivers had recently committed suicide. The drivers also were very aware of a number of student suicides and wanted to know what they could do to help. The role of school personnel as outlined by Poland (1989a) was emphasized.

Crisis intervention training emphasized two key areas:

1. What to do in the case of an accident.
2. How to manage potential violent students.

The procedures to follow in case of an accident are outlined in Appendix A. The management of potentially violent students emphasized the basic strategies for intervention in a fight. Drivers were asked to think about two different intervention plans. First, what would they do if a fight broke out while the bus was parked at school? Second, what intervention is needed when the bus is en route when a fight breaks out? The second situation is much more difficult, as no other adults are readily available to assist. The drivers asked the transportation department to clarify what should be done. They asked the following questions:

1. When should we just let the students fight?
2. When should the bus pull off the road?
3. When should the students who are not fighting be evacuated from the bus?
4. When should the driver return to school to get help?

These are difficult questions to answer and need addressing by the transportation supervisor.

The driver-training project was very much appreciated by drivers.

The initial training was extended to all 440 drivers within a year. Several drivers wrote letters to the superintendent to show their appreciation. Drivers were paid their hourly wage to participate in the 4½-hour training. New drivers are in-serviced each August before they begin employment. Drivers are utilizing the information presented as evidenced by a driver last year who figured out who on her bus had written the suicide note and personally escorted her to the school counselor so assistance could be provided.

Thankfully, there have been no serious bus accidents since the training was implemented. There have been minor ones, and a coordinated team response involving the driver, transportation personnel, and the building crisis team has been found to be very helpful.

Bus safety programs for students are also provided regularly. A few elementary schools did not want early elementary students to see a film on bus safety because it left the audience to conclude that the bus had run over and killed a student. The transportation supervisor asked for our support to convince administrators that the film needed to be shown. We agreed with the supervisor that children must learn to be careful in bus loading zones. That is where the majority of bus deaths occur each year.

There is a movement now to screen bus drivers for drug and alcohol usage. This is a very positive step, but we also need to provide more training to bus drivers and need to recognize how difficult their job is. Schools need to consider putting two-way radios in all buses so that drivers can summon assistance.

The question of how to train bus drivers is a complex one. They need many skills, and districts should utilize existing personnel to in-service drivers in the same way that they in-service the staff that work inside the school building. Drivers should be included in the building and/or district crisis intervention planning. There are many examples of school bus accidents and tragedies that we could cite. We chose the following examples that illustrate prior planning and prevention:

1. Boy, 9, leads 34 to safety as bus burns (1987).
2. Worn school bus aides rescue team (1989).

DISTRICT AWARENESS OF CRISIS TEAMS

All district personnel need to be aware of the crisis plan. This includes clerical staff, aides, bus drivers, and maintenance staff. Including these staff members in annual in-service days allows time for discussion when pressure and stress are minimal.

Public Awareness

As reports and quite probably experiences with school-related violence or crises multiply, community residents usually begin to express more concern. Questions that frequently come up include:

1. Why are our schools becoming unsafe?
2. What is being done to control crime, violence, and other crises?
3. Why isn't good, old-fashioned discipline enough to control these situations?

When crises occur in the schools, the first question the community generally has is "What are you going to do about it?" Proactive planning in the case of crisis or disaster is usually a real PR plus. Articles can be submitted to local newspapers, community groups, etc., detailing the efforts a district has put into developing a crisis intervention plan, together with information that relates directly to productive ways for the community to interact with or support the school's efforts in the event of a crisis. General policies can be shared with PTOs and other community organizations.

SCHOOL SERVICES IN THE CONTEXT OF COMMUNITY SERVICES

It makes sense to consider "the big picture" in considering provision of crisis prevention programs. School services are almost without exception limited to school hours. Mental health professionals working in the schools can expect to be confronted with crises occurring at all hours of the day or night. We have found, for various reasons, that Friday afternoons at 3:30 are frequent times of crisis. Instead of overreacting (taking on crisis cases after hours) and virtually assuring burnout or underreacting (and minimizing the incident), it is important to determine in advance where and when incidents will be referred to community agencies.

A great deal of homework should be done (ideally by the crisis team counseling liaison) regarding the resources of your community. Educators, of course, cannot be equipped to diagnose and treat the multitude of problems that cross their paths, but they can certainly participate in a comprehensive system through observing behavior, assessing warning signs, and referring.

Elements of a comprehensive community crisis service should include several basic elements regardless of the organizational model (Hoff,

1978). These are 24-hour telephone service, face-to-face walk-in crisis service, emergency medical or psychiatric service, and linkage with established community emergency services such as police, rescue squads, food organizations, etc.

It is probably a very unusual community that offers all of these services. What's more, it is usually unrealistic, if not impossible for most communities to administer most of these services through a single agency. Unfortunately, in our experience it is far more common that each of these services with in the community operates in isolation from each other rather than in synchronicity.

Piecing together what is available and maintaining such information to date is a big job and an important function. What is more, as specified in Chapter 2, it is important to understand other community mental health functions, including grounds for admission to charity and private hospitals, processes involved in obtaining a mental illness warrant, commitment procedures, the juvenile justice system, and child protective services.

Sample District- and Community-Wide Comprehensive Crisis Programs

Across the country schools are formulating crisis management plans, and in some states it has become mandatory. One project was begun in Quakertown, Pennsylvania Community School District in 1984. It was modeled after the employee assistance programs established by business and industry. The overall approach involved early identification, intervention, referral, and follow-up of students at high risk who were evidencing warning signs. The crisis situations involved included physical abuse, sexual abuse, neglect, eating disorders, pregnancy, depression, major psychiatric illness, alcohol and drug abuse or overdose, suicide, truancy, and dropout.

A Student Assistance Core Team (coordinator, teacher, nurse, guidance counselor, building-level administrator, district-level administrator) developed guidelines for referral and intervention. Experts from the community came to the schools to provide ongoing specialized training across the areas, and the team was called on to "respond to student dysfunctional and/or self-destructive behaviors, and consider appropriate punitive measures together with appropriate helping measures."

Another "big-picture" approach was advocated by the Minnesota Department of Education in a proposal issued early in 1987 for the state legislature to implement a "whole-child" policy for serving high-risk students of every age. The proposal approaches the problems by involving parents and school personnel more effectively and also by strengthening ties to community resources: human welfare, public health, the justice system, and economic security. The statement notes that "Education should provide leadership in this partnership and be "a key facilitator of programs and services for at-risk learners when the objective is to alleviate barriers to learning." By late 1987, the state legislature enacted 10 new laws with student-at-risk orientation.

A comprehensive, multiagency program was also developed by Arlington County Public Schools in Virginia and entitled the *High-Risk Identification and Intervention Project*. In addition to dealing with procedures for more traditional emergencies, the administration aimed to expand their program to address two distinct areas. One involved the number of individual crises that appear to be a product of "modern" times: child suicides, drug abuse, bomb threats, terrorist attacks, etc. The other stressed the need to work together with the numerous community agencies and institutions to provide invaluable expertise and resources for dealing with crises and for providing support for "at-risk" students. The efforts involved three major activities:

1. Education. Administration and staff were educated regarding the signs and symptoms of high-risk students and conducted an information awareness agenda aimed at the "at-risk" student groups themselves.
2. Guidelines for management of emergencies when they do occur, together with how to access assessment and follow-up services within the school system.
3. Procedures for referring students to community mental health services, hospitals, or private practitioners.

A consulting team was on call to all schools within the district and also to special education facilities. Activities for consultation and training also occurred at the individual campus level.

CONCLUSIONS

"It's my suspicion that we are just at the beginning of a long road that will lead to safer schools" (Timpane, quoted by Jennings, 1989, p. 27). The number and variety of crisis situations that impact on the schools appear to be at a record high. Numerous statistics have been presented to document that fact. There has been a historical lack of preparation for crises in the schools. Crises can occur in any size school or any neighborhood. Most school personnel have received no training in this area. Schools try to ignore crisis situations or respond spontaneously to manage the best they can. We also were unprepared for the crisis situations that we have faced in the schools, and this book is written to provide both a practical guide to crisis intervention and motivation for administrators, nurses, counselors, psychologists, and social workers to develop crisis plans.

Stevens (1990) stressed that schools get caught with their plans down, and administrators must get more savvy about crisis intervention. Sadly, most crisis intervention efforts begin after the tragedy had occurred. Schools need to look at their personnel and organize crisis teams. Everyone must know his or her role. The crisis intervention model developed by Caplan (1964) provides an excellent theoretical model for schools to use. Schools especially need to emphasize the primary prevention level. What can be done to prevent the crisis from occurring? The following newspaper headlines are our favorites because they are examples of prior planning and prevention:

- Boy 9, leads 34 to safety as bus burns (1987).
- Worn school bus aides rescue team (1989).
- Teacher's foresight helps class scare off suspect (1987).
- Dade teaches kids to say no to gun: First graders savvy about weapons (1989).
- Students offer peers safe ride home (1990).
- Educators learn the science of gangs (Jones, 1991).
- Stiff federal law highlighted to fight guns, drugs in schools (Markley, 1991b).
- 13 schools seek out weapons with metal detectors (Markley, 1991c).
- Campus crime prompts vigilance: Parents students link up for safety (Markley, 1991a).
- Youngsters learn to settle conflicts without violence (1991).

We wish that we had located hundreds of clippings that illustrate preventive efforts.

There will undoubtedly be more legislation such as the Right to Safe Schools Constitutional Amendment that passed in California in 1982. Administrators will be faced with increasing legal questions about their role in keeping schools safe. Several authors have stressed the need for closer coordination between the schools and the judicial system. We heartily support that recommendation. The schools must learn to work more closely with all community resources and agencies. Those who commit crimes at school must receive consequences and assistance from all possible sources. The National School Safety Center* is an invaluable resource to the public schools. We hope that we are indeed on course for schools that are prepared for crisis situations. The importance of participation and prior planning cannot be overemphasized. An oft-cited biblical quote illustrates this point: "I must work the works of Him that sent me, while it is day: the night cometh when no man can work" (Gospel of St. John, Chapter 9, Verse 4). The time for crisis planning is today, while things are normal in your particular school. Crisis intervention is, according to Stevens (1990), an inside job that begins with a prepared staff and involves the students and the community. The response of the schools must be an active one. If a crisis can not be prevented, schools must mobilize quickly to assist the victims. Those trying to assist, such as counselors and psychologists, must seek out the student victims and work with them and their parents.

*The NSSC publishes resource papers, workbooks, and guidelines on school safety. They also distribute excellent films on school safety issues. Their address is: 4165 Thousand Oaks Boulevard, Suite 290, Westlake Village, California 91362. Their phone number is (805) 373-9977.

APPENDIX A

Possible Responsibilities for Crisis Team Members at Primary, Secondary, and Tertiary Levels of Prevention

CAMPUS LIAISON/COORDINATOR

Characteristics

This individual must be able to organize and make decisions during the crisis. Someone with authority to make policy decisions is a necessity. This individual should also be familiar with superiors within the school district and the political role the district plays in the community. Usually an administrator such as a principal or assistant superintendent is appropriate for this role.

Primary Prevention Activities

1. Take responsibility for the establishment, coordination, and clarification of tasks for the crisis team members in each building.
2. Establish communication lines to district central administration and establish exactly what information will be communicated and how during an emergency. For example, in one district an emergency message flashes across the computer screens of all schools in the district when a crisis or disaster has occurred at another building. In this manner phone lines are not tied up, and communication can continue. Backup systems for communication despite electrical failure, phone outage, etc., should also be established.
3. Establish communication lines and coordination policy with any organized community crisis or disaster teams that may become involved.

4. Convene meetings of crisis team and help to coordinate any crisis drills that need to occur.
5. Establish a "second in command" in case this individual is not in the building during a crisis.

Secondary Prevention Activities

1. Alert team members of a crisis.
2. Make decisions regarding changing class schedules, securing the building, issuing directives or announcements over the intercom system.
3. Communicate with central administration and community disaster teams.
4. Coordinate activities of team members. Keep in touch with all members to do so.
5. Make decisions regarding possible courses of action when necessary.
6. Provide for meeting of crisis team following the crisis or at appropriate intervals during the crisis. A "cool-down" meeting following each day to provide support for each other and to exchange information should be arranged.
7. As far as is possible, keep records of what has been done and what factual information is available regarding the incident. Put this in writing for dissemination to teachers, parents, and media at the earliest possible point.

Tertiary Prevention Activities

1. Provide long-term assistance and support to campus personnel as needed.

PARENT LIAISON

Characteristics

The selected individual should be comfortable speaking before a large group and have skills to manage highly emotional reactions in parents both individually and in groups. A highly visible individual whom the parents already know and deal with on a regular basis appears to be the most comforting in times of crisis. One of the best ways to help children who experience a crisis is to help their parents. This is not the place for a consultant.

Primary Prevention Activities

1. Educate parents regarding the existence of the school crisis plan, its objectives, and the necessity for it.
2. Develop a relationship with parents so that they feel they know and trust their school contact person. This should reduce panic resulting from wild rumors that are often associated with crisis events.

3. Develop materials that may be needed for the dissemination of information at the time of a disaster or crisis. Keep them in a handy, "ready-to-go" place. These materials should include:
   a. A draft of a letter to parents informing them of what has happened and when and how they should contact the school for further information. This might include the time and date of the first public meeting or discussion.
   b. Information regarding how to work with and talk with their children following a tremendous shock and what to expect in themselves.
   c. How the school district intends to manage the situation. It is important to make sure the parents are aware of all of the district efforts to protect, support, and comfort children.
4. Develop a list of referrals for private counseling at all levels of ability to pay. Have this typed into a form that may be handed out to parents.
5. Identify parents who live near the school who are available to help in a crisis. Schedule a rehearsal meeting and clarify how they can assist.

Secondary Prevention Activities

In the event of a crisis or disaster:
1. Provide parents with information regarding exactly what is known to have happened.
2. Implement the plan to manage the phone calls and parents who arrive at the school, if necessary.
3. Schedule and attend an open question-and-answer meeting for parents as soon after the incident as possible.

Tertiary Prevention Activities

1. Implement follow-up meetings with parents. These meetings may occur for weeks or even months following a disaster. Parents may be invited to continuing "update" meetings to follow their concerns over time.
2. Gather feedback from parents, staff, and fellow crisis team members to determine if the plans were effective. Incorporate suggestions for improvements into preparation for future crises.

Sample Materials

*Helping Your Child in a Crisis or Disaster**

It is common for children to regress behaviorally and academically during crises. Parents need both to provide structure and to be patient. Children and adolescents have pronounced reactions to crises or disaster shortly following the event and for some time to follow. A constructive way to view the situation is that they are normal children in an abnormal circumstance (a major stressor or disaster).

*From Farberow and Gordon (1981).

Most of the emotional problems that come up can be attributed to stress and can be expected to be fairly brief. After your child has experienced some relief and comfort together with some time to get over the stress, the chances are that he or she will readjust well. Support and understanding at the family level is the first, and many times the most powerful, resource for helping children. This pamphlet should, however, provide you as parents with some general information that we hope will answer your questions regarding your child's reaction and readjustment to this tragedy. The following are common emotional and behavioral reactions among children:

Fears and Worries.   It is natural for children to have serious concerns and fears following a disaster or crisis. Remember it is often the parent's reaction that determines how quickly they recover from the shock they are going through. It is generally best to accept the child's fears as being very real to him or to her, even if they sound unrealistic or unwarranted to you. Your child will need some extra support and some time. It may be necessary to treat him or her as if he or she were a couple of years younger until he or she readjusts: more naps, more hugs, holding, and thumb-sucking may reemerge; he or she may have more difficulty controlling his or her temper or teary reactions; and he or she may become more clinging and demanding of your time.

Denial.   It is fairly common for children, adolescents, and adults to have difficulty accepting a suddenly changed reality. For example, a child may insist on returning to a house when it has been destroyed, or an adolescent may insist that his or her friend will be fine when the friend is in a coma and about to die. This is the individual's way of expressing that the circumstance is simply too overwhelming to manage at that time. The reality should be gently but firmly pointed out to the individual. Although he or she might become angry, arguments should be avoided. Eventually the shock will wear off, and that person will accept the reality if given the time, support, and clear messages of what has occurred. When there is a prolonged or intense period of denial, the remainder of the grieving process may be somewhat prolonged or especially upsetting to the child. He or she may go through very angry periods, very tearful, depressed periods, and/or briefer reoccurrences of denial before finally reaching a phase of calm acceptance of what has happened.

Sleep Disturbances; Acting Younger Than Chronological Age.   Problems with sleeping are among the most common reactions of children to a disaster or crisis. They may fear going to bed or going to bed alone. Often children make requests to sleep with their parents or siblings or to have a light burning. Nightmares or refusal to go to sleep for long periods may require professional intervention. It may be necessary to support the child around bedtime issues for a few weeks or months. It might help to stay with your child until he or she falls asleep. A regular bedtime routine that you may have used when he or she was younger may be comforting. Evening activities that are calming and restful may prepare the child, together with the old standard of a cup of warm milk.

At times children begin to wet the bed at night following a shock or a crisis.

Loss of bowel or bladder control is fairly common, even if she or he has not had such accidents in years. If this does occur, it is important to be understanding about it and to avoid embarrassment or harassment to the child. Like the other symptoms, this pattern should disappear as your child adjusts to the shock.

School Avoidance and School Phobia. Following a major shock children often fer leaving their families and loved ones. Going to school, especially if there have been anxieties about school in the past, may become a problem. It is important to communicate to your child that, no matter what, he or she must go to school. It is an important part of his or her life with peers and necessary toward the development of independence. Often children will point out aspects of the school or staff that they fear; however, in almost every case, it is the fear of leaving home that is really behind the school phobia. It may be necessary to confer with the child's teacher and counselor to develop a supportive plan with which to ease the child's adjustment to returning to or continuing to attend school.

Help for Your Child

1. Talk with your child about what has happened; provide as much information as you feel he or she can understand.
2. Allow your child to express and label his or her emotions.
3. Allow your child to grieve or verbalize his or her concerns over the loss of a lost relationship, toy, or other significant object or opportunity.
4. Reassure your child that things will work out and that you are together. He or she may need this assurance again and again.
5. Hold your child, pat your child, and hug your child more often than you ordinarily might.
6. Spend some "special" time with your child alone each day. Good times include just before bed, after dinner, or after a nap.
7. Provide opportunities for movement-oriented games and lots of gross motor activities. Tension and anxieties can be relieved through physical activity.
8. You may want to contact your child's teacher and try to help with any difficulties—behavioral, motivational, or concentration problems she or he may be experiencing in the classroom.
9. You may contact _____ at the following numbers for more information regarding children's reactions to crisis or to discuss further help.

Symptoms of Reaction to Crisis or Disaster in Adults*

First Reactions

1. Numbness, shock, difficulty believing what has happened or is in the process of happening. Physical and mental reactions may be very slow or confused.

*From Farberow and Frederick (1981).

2. Difficulty in decision making. It may be difficult to settle on a course of action or to make even small judgment calls. You may feel uncertain about just about everything for a while.

Ongoing Reactions

1. Loss of appetite, difficulty sleeping, loss of interest or pleasure in everyday activities.
2. Desire to get away from everyone. Finding company of others unpleasant, even friends and family.
3. Emotional lability. You may find yourself quite irritable and react with anger or tears much more quickly than normally.
4. Emotional, physical, and mental feelings of fatigue, hopelessness, and helplessness. You may feel physically ill or experience increased numbers of headaches, stomach problems, or backaches.
5. Children may be more clinging, unhappy, and needy of parental attention and comfort. This creates increased tension, and your impulse to hit or be short with children may be stronger. More child abuse and marital discord follow adjustments to major crisis or disaster.
6. It may be difficult to accept that the crisis or disaster had any impact on you or to accept support from your friends and community.

Some Things That Can Be Helpful

1. Take time to relax and do things you find pleasant. Getting away for a few hours with close friends is often helpful.
2. Try to avoid making changes until you have adjusted. Stick with your regular routine, your regular bank, your regular job, and schedule. Any change creates stress, even if it is a positive one.
3. Remember any of the feelings you just read about above are normal reactions to crisis or disaster and will subside with time. If you are able to discuss them with friends or family, they may subside more quickly.
4. Get regular exercise or participate in a regular sport. Activity soothes anxiety and helps you to relax.
5. Get some information and develop a plan regarding how you and your spouse will talk to and support your children.
6. Keep your sense of humor and appreciate the positive side of your situation as much as possible. Remind yourself that this will be easier to do as time goes on.

TEACHER LIAISON

Characteristics

This individual will be most effective if he or she is generally known, liked, and trusted by the staff. A building-level assistant principal or counselor is a likely position. This individual must have a schedule that permits him or her to leave the routine job for hours at a time without seriously disrupting the students' day.

Primary Prevention Activities

1. Materials development
   a. Handout for teachers regarding what behavioral/emotional reactions to expect from their students.
   b. Handout for teachers regarding the sorts of classroom activities and materials that might be appropriate following the crisis.
   c. Instructions for teachers as to how to identify children who should be sent out of class and those who should not. If children are to be sent from class under some circumstances, be sure to specify where and, if necessary, what periods of the day. (This will probably require consultation with the crisis team counseling liaison.)
1. Educate teachers regarding the existence of a crisis team and the general plan to manage future crises. Consider some of these general policies:
   a. A universal cue or code word might be established to surreptitiously alert teaching staff to do the following:
      i. "Freeze" the schedule and keep the present class until further notice.
      ii. Close and possibly lock classroom doors.
      iii. Meet after school for further information.
      iv. Evacuate the building (usually the fire alarm). Policies need to be established that can operate as a backup to intercom inaccessibility or in spite of electrical failure.
   b. Each teacher should have an established method for contacting the office in case of a classroom emergency. Some methods might include sending a student with various colors of construction paper: green for minor emergency—need help when convenient; yellow for moderate emergency—someone should come to the classroom immediately; and red for severe emergencies that require the immediate attention of several adults.
   c. The teaching staff should be aware who their crisis team contact person is and how and when information will be disseminated to them. One standard expectation is that the teaching staff will meet at the finish of any day in which a crisis has occurred right after school at a certain location.

Secondary Prevention Activities

1. Issue instructions to the teachers, possibly in terms of codes over the intercom.

2. Arrange and attend a "debriefing" period for teachers immediately after school.
   a. All known information should be given to teaching staff, and a plan for the following day should be discussed.
   b. Materials developed for suggested classroom activities and what symptoms to expect in students should be passed out as appropriate.
   c. Review protocol for sending students out of class.
   d. Provide emotional support, praise, and encouragement.
   e. Screen for teachers who appear to be having a great deal of difficulty coping with the crisis. Consider extra personnel to help or even temporarily to replace personnel who appear likely to exacerbate the crisis.
   f. Consider meeting with staff part way through the following day to offer them an opportunity to vent and to discuss how the plan is working out. Certainly meet with staff at the close of the following day and days after as is necessary. Some crises may require weekly meetings for a month after.
3. Immediately following the crisis circulate in the building to speak with teachers as much as is possible. Personal contact is often a great source of support.

Tertiary Prevention Activities

1. Meet with teachers and crisis team to process how the plan went and to modify basic procedures as needed.

Sample Materials

Tips for Teachers in Dealing with Crisis

There have been many varied crisis situations that have impacted the school. There will be occasions when administrators, counselors and psychologists can not provide immediate assistance to all who need it during a crisis. Teachers can provide very valuable assistance. The goal of crisis intervention is to provide immediate assistance to restore normalcy and minimize debilitating lasting effects.

Verification

Your principal will verify the extent of the crisis and notify you as soon as possible. Please be very cautious about commenting to students until you are notified of the facts. Tell students that it is important to stay calm and that rumors can get out of hand and that you will give them the facts as soon as possible.

Our Crisis Reaction

Reaction to a crisis can fall into the categories of panic or defeat. It is normal to have lots of anxiety and to want to flee the scene or to feel that the world is not a very secure place. Unresolved issues based on our life history may surface and add to our emotional state. Waves of emotions may flood our thoughts.
What Can the Teacher Do?

1. After receiving verification from the principal you should openly and honestly acknowledge what has happened. Students need to be told the facts in age appropriate terms. This will help de-escalate the situation.
2. Model expression of your feelings and give the students permission to express their feelings. By giving permission to express feelings, they become validated leading to return to normalcy more quickly.
3. It is important that students understand that they may be flooded with waves of emotion and there is not one correct way to feel. Our emotions range through these stages and we can go back and forth through them.
4. Following the crisis, be alert for those students who are experiencing more extreme reactions in comparison to the norm and refer them to the appropriate counselor.
5. Once students are physically safe they need the opportunity to talk out feelings concerning having their safety and security threatened.
6. We have a tendency to expect all students to react to bad news with feelings of remorse. Give permission for a range of emotions and recognize the student who says today "I don't care or it doesn't bother me" may be crying tomorrow or next week. Students may show their feelings through "acting out" behaviors.
7. Provide opportunities for students who wish to do so to express thoughts through their writing.
8. Be prepared to provide follow-up discussions as needed in the future or as more information about the crisis may last a long time.

Dealing with Death

A death in the school family (either a student or faculty member) is difficult. Statistics indicate that as many as 1 out of every 750 students die or are killed each year. The life event history of each person will have a great deal to do with the ability to cope with a death in the school family.

1. Tell students about death in a quiet and direct manner.
2. Avoid religious platitudes and recognize the varying religious beliefs held by students.
3. Give permission for a range of emotions.
4. Do not offer unnecessary details but do answer all questions.

5. Physical contact may comfort some students.
6. Discuss the meaning and effect of the loss and discuss funeral etiquette, and appropriate memorials or remembrances of the deceased.

Classroom Activities*

Many of the teachers have responded to disasters with creative classroom activities to support their students in ventilating and getting over their shocking experience. Maybe these ideas will serve as "springboards" for your own and/or could be adapted to meet your own students' needs.

Preschool Activities

1. Availability of toys that encourage play reenactment of a child's experiences and observations during the disaster can be helpful to him or her in integrating these experiences. These might include fire trucks, dump trucks, rescue trucks, ambulances, building blocks, or puppets or dolls as ways for the child to ventilate his or her own feelings about what has occurred.

2. Children need lots of physical contact during times of stress to help them reestablish ego boundaries and a sense of security. Games that involve physical touching among children within a structure are helpful in this regard. Some examples might be Ring Around the Rosie, London Bridge, or Duck, Duck, Goose.

3. Providing extra amounts of finger foods in small portions and fluids is a concrete way of supplying the emotional and physical nourishment children need in times of stress. Oral satisfaction is especially necessary, as children tend to revert to more regressive behavior in response to feeling that their survival or security is threatened.

4. Have the children do a mural on butcher paper with topics such as what happened in your house (school or neighborhood) when the big storm (earthquate, etc.) hit. This is recommended for small groups with discussion afterward facilitated by an adult.

5. "Short stories" dictated to an adult on an one-to-one basis on such topics as "What I do and don't like about _____." This activity can help the children verbalize their fears as well as perhaps get them back in touch with previous positive associations with the disruptive phenomena.

6. Have the children draw pictures about the disaster and then discuss the pictures in small groups. The activity allows them to vent their experiences and to discover that others share their fears.

7. Do a group collage.

8. In small groups have each child take a turn at answering the question, "If you were an animal, what would you be, and what would you do if it started raining hard?" This can be a nonthreatening way for children to express their

*From Lystad (1985).

fears. The adult might end each turn by having the children tell how they would make themselves safe as a child rather than as an animal.

Primary School Activities

1. For the younger children, availability of toys that encourage play reenactment of their experiences and observations during the disaster can be helpful in their integrating these experiences. These might include ambulances, dump trucks, fire trucks, building blocks, and dolls. Play with puppets can provide ways for older children, as well, to ventilate their feelings and reactions.

2. Help or encourage the children to develop skits or puppet shows about what happened in the disaster. Encourage them to include anything positive about the experience as well as those aspects that were frightening or disconcerting.

3. Do a group mural on butcher paper with topics such as "What happened in your neighborhood (school or home) when _____." This is recommended for small groups with discussion afterward, facilitated by an adult. It can help children feel less isolated with their fears and provide the opportunity to vent their feelings.

4. Have the children create short stories (written or dictated to an adult, depending on their ages) about their experience in the disaster.

5. Have the children draw pictures and then talk about them in small groups on such topics as: (1) What happened when the disaster hit? (2) How did you help your family during the disaster? (3) How could you help your parents if you were in another disaster? How can we be prepared for a disaster? (4) Did anything good happen during the storm? (5) What did you, or anyone you know, lose during the disaster? It is important in the group discussion to end on a positive note, that is, a feeling of mastery or preparedness, noting that the community or family pulled together to deal with the crisis, etc., as well as to provide a vehicle for expressing their feelings about what took place.

6. Stimulate group discussion about disaster experiences by showing your own feelings, fears, or experiences during the flood. It is very important to legitimize their feelings and to help them feel less isolated.

7. Have the children brainstorm on their own classroom or family disaster plan. What would they do? What would they take if they had to evacuate? How would they contact parents? How should the family be prepared? How could they help the family? Encourage them to discuss these things with their families.

8. Encourage class activities in which children can *organize* or *build* projects (scrapbooks, replicas, etc.), thus giving them a sense of mastery and ability to organize what seem like chaotic and confusing events.

9. Encourage "disaster" games in which children set rules and develop outcomes that can allow them to develop feelings of mastery over events.

10. Have the children color the pictures in "The Awful Rain and How It Made Me Feel" (or similar material appropriate to the disaster). *Encourage the children to talk about their own feelings* during and after the disaster.

Junior High and High School Activities

1. Group discussion of their experiences of the disaster is particularly important among adolescents. They need the opportunity to vent as well as to normalize the extreme emotions that come up for them. A good way to stimulate such a
discussion is for the teacher to share her or his own reactions to the disaster.
Adolescents may need considerable reassurance that even extreme emotions and
"crazy thoughts" are normal in a disaster. It is important to end such discussions
on a positive note (e.g., What heroic acts were observed? How can we be of help
at home or in the community? How could we be more prepared for a disaster?).
Such discussion is appropriate for any course of study in that it can facilitate a
return to more normal functioning.

2. Break the class into small groups and have them develop a disaster plan for
their home, school, or community. This can be helpful in repairing a sense of
mastery and security as well as having practical merit. The small groups might
then share their plans in a discussion with the entire class. Encourage students to
share their plans with their families. They may wish to conduct a "family disaster
preparedness" meeting and invite family members and disaster preparedness
experts to participate.

3. Conduct a class discussion and/or support a class project on how the
students might help the community rehabilitation effort. It is important to help
them develop concrete and realistic ways to be of assistance. This helps them to
overcome the feelings of helplessness, frustration, and "survivor's guilt" that are
common in disaster situations.

4. Classroom activities that relate the disaster to course study can be a good
way to help the students integrate their own experience or observations while
providing specific learning experiences. In implementing the following suggestions (or similar ideas of your own) *it is very important to allow time for the students to
discuss feelings that are stimulated by the projects or issues covered.*

Journalism. Have the students write stories that cover different aspects of the
disaster. These might include community impact, lawsuits that result from
disaster, human interest stories from fellow students, geological impact, etc.
Issues such as an accurate reporting of catastrophic events verses one with
sensationalist overtones might be discussed. The stories might be compiled into a
special student publication.

Science. Cover scientific aspects of the disaster: discuss climatic conditions, geological impact, etc. Have a project about stress: cover physiological responses to
stress and methods of dealing with it. Discuss how flocks of birds and herds of
animals band together and work in a threatening or emergency situation. What
can be learned from their instinctive actions?

English Composition. Have the students write about their own experiences in the
disaster. Such issues as the problems that arise in conveying heavy emotional
tone without being overly dramatic might be discussed.

Literature. Have students report on natural disasters in Greek mythology, American and British literature, and in poetry.

Psychology. Have the students apply what they have learned in the course to the emotions, behaviors, and stress reactions they felt or observed in the disaster. Cover posttraumatic stress syndrome. Have a guest speaker from the mental health professions involved in disaster work with victims, etc. Have students discuss (from their own experience) what things have been most helpful in assisting them to deal with disaster-related stress. Have students develop a mental health education brochure that discusses emotional/behavioral reactions to disaster-related stress. Have students conduct a survey among their parents or friends: "What was the most dangerous situation in which you ever found yourself?" "How did you react psychologically?"

Peer Counseling. Provide special information on common responses to disaster; encourage the students' helping each other to integrate their own experiences.

Health. Discuss emotional reactions to disaster, the importance of taking care of one's own emotional and physical well-being, etc. Discuss health implications of the disaster, such as water contamination, food that may have gone bad because of the lack of refrigeration, and other health precautions and safety measures. Discuss the effects of adrenalin on the body during the stress and the danger. A guest speaker from a local public health and/or mental health organization might be invited to the class.

Art. Have the students portray their experiences of the disaster in various art media. This may be done individually or as a group effort (e.g., making a mural).

Speech/Drama. Have the students portray the catastrophic emotions that come up in response to a disaster. Have them develop a skit or play on some aspects of the event. Conduct a debate: Resolved that women are more psychologically prepared to handle stress than men (or vice versa).

Math. Have the class solve mathematical problems related to the impact of the disaster (e.g., build questions around gallons of water lost, cubic feet of earth that moved in a mud slide).

Civics/Government. Study governmental agencies responsible for aid to victims, how they work, how effective they are, and their political implications within a community. Examine the community systems and how the stress of the disaster has affected them. Have students invite a local governmental official to class to discuss disaster precautions, warning systems, etc. Have students contact the legislators regarding recent disaster-related bills passed or pending. How will this legislation affect your community and other areas of the state? Visit local emergency operating centers and learn about their functioning.

History. Have students report on natural disasters that have occurred in your community or geographic area and the lessons that were learned that can be useful in preparing for future disasters.

When to Refer to the Counselor (Psychologist)

Following a disaster, children and adolescents display a number of different "symptoms" that are quite normal. Most of your students will respond to support from you and their families over time. Under some circumstances, however, additional counseling may be needed. Students who were easily upset historically, who have lost close family members or are from historically unstable families, or students at high risk for crisis in general are the most likely to require additional help following a disaster. Please refer students to the counselor's office:

1. If the student is extremely tearful or emotional, cannot begin to be involved with classroom activities, and does not respond to comfort or support.
2. If the reactions considered to be "normal" do not diminish over a period of months.
3. If the student is very withdrawn or depressed and does not respond to comfort or support.

Older children (junior high or high school) may exhibit other behaviors that should be referred on immediately:

1. If the student seems to be confused about who he or she is, who people he or she knows well are, what day or time it is, and where he or she is when in a known place.
2. If he or she talks of wanting to hurt or kill him- or herself or someone else, or if he or she mutilates him- or herself (for example, cutting forearm or scratching self until bleeding).
3. If he or she appears to be using drugs or alcohol excessively, and this pattern is uncommon for the student.
4. If he or she stops caring for personal hygiene and loses or gains a significant amount of weight.
5. If he or she begins to have times during which he or she sees, hears, or smells things that aren't there (hallucinations); receives "messages" from outer space, the television or radio; or is fancifully convinced that someone is after him or trying to hurt him or her.
6. If speech becomes very fast and somewhat nonsensical, he or she cannot sit down, flies off the handle easily, and/or gets "wild ideas."

Caring for the Caretaker

When working with those experiencing crises it is important to recognize that, to some extent, this places you in crisis too. The demands of this work are intense and never ending. We don't want you to burn out. Please watch out for the beginning signs, which are:

1. *Emotionally,* feeling sad, hopeless, helpless, as if you "just don't care" any more.
2. *Physically,* having little energy, stomach pains, headaches, eating too much or too little, sleeping too much or too little, waking in the middle of the night or early morning hours.
3. *Mentally,* having difficulty concentrating, feeling "mentally" too tired to organize your workload, losing objectivity in evaluating your own functioning or external confusion.

It is very important to notice these patterns in yourself. The more you feel free to vent your frustrations, feelings, and reactions with those you work with, the better you are likely to feel. If enough informal opportunities are not available to do this through the course of the day, it may be necessary to set aside times for everyone to get together, have lunch, and chat or gripe about your experiences.

Teaching under the best of circumstances is a stressful profession. It is "normal" that under disaster or crisis conditions, when you are managing your own personal reaction together with those of your students, at times it will feel overwhelming. Everyone is strongly encouraged to take care of him- or herself by taking the following steps:

1. Don't take on any new school projects or extra work at school. Just keep your day as simple as possible.
2. Have students or assistants correct papers, take care of duplicating, or manage other time-consuming tasks. Choose your lessons with this in mind.
3. Do as many "whole-class" activities as possible. This cuts down on lesson plans and discipline problems.
4. Set aside time at the end of the day, or if necessary twice each day (before lunch and before going home), to do special "fun" things. Students can work for this by behaving properly. This cuts down on the number of times you may need to reprimand students.
5. Take time to discuss the event and compare personal reactions with the other members of the staff who were involved in the experience.

COUNSELING/STUDENT LIAISON

Characteristics

This individual must be familiar with student emotional needs and be proficient in basic counseling techniques for crisis and disasters. It is necessary that this individual be able to work in tandem with the teacher and parent liaison team members to prevent as many severe emotional reactions as possible.

Primary Prevention Activities

Institute routine educational programs for children and adolescents that might prevent crises: drug abuse prevention programs, sexual abuse prevention programs, and teaching of coping skills in the classroom.

Secondary Prevention Activities

1. Plan ways of using community resources that would be easily accessed during an emergency. These will include mental health agency personnel, clergy, and professionals within the school district.
2. Train any paraprofessionals in basic psychological first aid, basic crisis counseling, and recognition of symptoms associated with mild to severe emotional reactions.

Tertiary Prevention Activities

1. Follow up counseling and or monitoring of affected students.
2. Assist students with community or school rehabilitation projects.

Sample Materials

*Reactions of Children to Disaster**

Typical reactions for children of all ages include:

- Fears of future disasters.
- Loss of interest in school.
- Regressive behavior.
- Sleep disturbance and night terrors.
- Fears of natural events associated with the disaster.

Different age groups of children tend to be vulnerable to the stress of disaster in unique ways. Below, typical responses are summarized for various age groups and suggested responses to them.

Preschool (Ages 1–5)

Typical responses in this age group include thumb-sucking, bed-wetting, fears of the darkness or animals, clinging to parents, night terrors, loss of bladder or bowel control, constipation, speech difficulties (e.g., stammering), and loss of or

*From Farberow and Gordon (1981).

increase of appetite. Children in this age group are particularly vulnerable to disruption of their previously secure world. Because they generally lack the verbal and conceptual skills necessary to cope effectively with sudden stress by themselves, they look to family members for comfort. They are often strongly affected by the reactions of parents and other family members. Abandonment is a major fear in this age group, and children who have lost family members or even pets or toys will need special reassurance.

The goals of the following suggestions are to help the child to integrate his or her experiences and to reestablish a sense of security and mastery:

- Encourage expression through play reenactment.
- Provide verbal reassurance and physical comforting.
- Give frequent attention.
- Encourage expression regarding loss of pets or toys.
- Provide comforting bedtime routines.
- Allow child to sleep in same room with parents (with the understanding that this is for a limited period of time).

Early Childhood (Ages 5–11)

Common responses in this age group include:

- Irritability.
- Whining.
- Clinging.
- Aggressive behavior at home or school.
- Overt competition with younger siblings for parents' attention.
- Night terrors, nightmares, fear of darkness.
- School avoidance.
- Withdrawal from peers.
- Loss of interest and poor concentration in school.

Regressive behavior is most typical of this group. Loss of pets and prized objects is particularly difficult for them to handle. The following responses may be helpful:

- Patience and tolerance.
- Play sessions with adults and peers.
- Discussions with adults and peers.
- Relaxation of expectations in school or at home (with clear understanding that this is temporary and that the normal routine will be resumed after a time).
- Opportunities for structured but not demanding chores and responsibilities at home.
- Rehearsal of safety measures to be taken in future crises or disasters.

Preadolescent (Ages 11–14)

Common responses in this age group are:

- Sleep disturbance.
- Appetite disturbance.
- Rebellion in the home.
- Refusal to do chores.
- School problems (e.g., fighting, withdrawal, loss of interest, attention-seeking behavior).
- Physical problems (e.g., headaches, vague aches and pains, skin eruptions, bowel problems, psychosomatic complaints).
- Loss of interest in peer social activities.

Peer reactions are especially significant in this age group. The child needs to feel that his or her fears are both appropriate and shared by others. Responses should be aimed at lessening tensions and anxieties and possible guilt feelings. The following may be helpful:

- Group activities geared toward the resumption of routines.
- Involvement with same-age-group activity.
- Group discussions geared toward reliving the disaster and rehearsing appropriate behavior in future disasters.
- Structured but undemanding responsibilities.
- Temporarily relaxed expectations of performance at school and at home.
- Additional individual attention and consideration.

Adolescent (Ages 14–18)

Common responses in this age group include:

- Psychosomatic symptoms (e.g., rashes, bowel problems, headaches, asthma).
- Appetite and sleep disturbance.
- Hypochondriasis.
- Amenorrhea or dysmenorrhea.
- Agitation or decrease in energy level; apathy.
- Decline in interest in the opposite sex.
- Irresponsible and/or delinquent behavior.
- Decline in emancipatory struggles over parent control.
- Poor concentration.

Most of the activities and interests of the adolescent are focused on her own and his own age peers. Adolescents tend to be especially distressed by the disruption of their peer-group activities and the lack of access to full adult responsibilities in community efforts.

The following responses are recommended:

- Encourage participation in the community rehabilitation or reclamation work.
- Encourage resumption of social activities, athletics, clubs, etc.
- Encourage discussion of disaster experiences with peers, extrafamily members, significant others.
- Temporarily reduce expectations for level of school and general performance.
- Encourage, but do not insist on, discussion of disaster fears within the family setting.

General Steps in the Helping Process*

A basic principle in working with problems of children in disasters is that they are essentially normal children who have experienced great stress. Most of the problems that appear are likely, therefore, to be directly related to the disaster and temporary.

The primary goal of crisis counseling is to identify, respond to, and relieve the stresses developed as a result of the crisis (disaster) and then to reestablish normal functioning as quickly as possible. Sometimes the reaction is mild; at other times it is severe.

The general steps in the helping process are:

1. Establishing rapport.
   a. Letting the children know you are interested in them and want to help them.
   b. Checking with the children to make sure that they understand what you are saying and that you understand them.
   c. Having genuine respect and regard for the children and their families.
   d. Communicating trust and promising only what you can do.
   e. Communicating acceptance of the children and their families.
   f. Communicating to the children and their families that you are an informed authority.
2. Identifying, defining, and focusing on the problem. Like adults, children going through a crisis may seem confused and chaotic in their thinking. It is helpful to the children and families to identify a specific problem, to define it, and to focus on it first. If possible, the problem should be quickly resolved so that the children and families quickly experience a sense of success and control. Evaluating the seriousness of the problem should determine the families' capacity for dealing with it.

*From Farberow and Gordon (1981).

3. Understanding feelings. Empathy is the ability to see and feel as others do. Being empathetic with children requires patience, for children frequently are unable to express their fears, and the adults need to appreciate the kind and intensity of the children's feelings. For example, adults may be required to listen to a child's account of a disaster many times while the child "works through" the disaster by talking it out.

4. Listening carefully. Frequently, the children's experiences of adults listening to them are unsatisfactory. In working with children, efforts should be made to respond to them and to comment frequently. Interrupting the children should be avoided, for it tends to happen often, and the children may be particularly sensitive to being interrupted by adults.

5. Communicating clearly. It is important to communicate in language the children understand. The presence of the family is useful in interviews with the children, for the families will be more familiar with them and their behavior. In addition, families will be able to learn how to communicate with the children better after observing the interviewer. Simple language should be used in speaking to the children so that they are not excluded from the helping process.

STUDENT LIAISON

Characteristics

An individual with knowledge of school administrative policies and some understanding of law enforcement.

Primary Prevention Activities

1. Assist students to begin such programs as Students Against Drunk Driving, Students Against Suicide, mediation.
2. Develop curriculum units on safety that address guns, automobiles, bicycles, etc.
3. Identify student leaders or assistants to help if a crisis occurs.

Secondary Prevention Activities

Utilize student leaders and assistance to help control students.

Tertiary Prevention Activities

Provide long-term assistance and support to students.

MEDIA LIAISON

Characteristics

This should be an individual who is comfortable with appearances on television and radio. Good interpersonal skills are absolutely necessary. This individual must also be assertive and able to set limits without offending the members of the press or the observing public. Since an understanding of the district's public policy in a broader sense is also desirable, it is often most pragmatic for this person to be an out-of-building, district-level individual. Positions such as an assistant superintendent work well.

Primary Prevention Activities

1. Acquire training in district public relations policy and limits for the media. In particular, the following questions must be answered:
   a. Will media be allowed to film or interview students inside the building? If so, under what circumstances?
   b. What information, if any, will be withheld from the media and under what circumstances (e.g., names, if family has not been notified; information that is not confirmed)?
   c. How will the district or building respond to questions to which the answers are not yet known?
2. Develop a general format for a "press release" or a written statement of what is known to have happened to release to the media.
3. As far as is possible, become familiar with radio/television channel's policies for broadcasting crisis information and the names of the contact people.

Secondary Prevention Activities

1. Report immediately to the scene of the crisis when summoned.
2. Respond to telephone calls from the media.
3. Greet and "contain" members of the media who may arrive on campus. Provide a room near the building entrance where media may discuss the incident.
4. Use the media coverage opportunity to communicate with community agencies and parents, if necessary. Thus, parents might be advised of altered bus schedules, class schedules, personnel changes, etc.
5. Serve as moderator and mediator for any other interview that may be granted to media (e.g., teachers, parents, students) in the building or on school grounds.
6. Consult with team coordinator's log of events to write a press release. Update the press release several times per day as more information becomes available.

Tertiary Prevention Activities

1. Review process and update methods for future.
2. Provide follow-up information to media relating:
   a. All information known in the final analysis.
   b. District's actions and management of the problem.
   c. Any updated plans for dealing with such future crises, especially if the district was caught somewhat unaware by the event (e.g., the Brown School District is planning to implement annual disaster drills so schools will be prepared for future emergencies).

MEDICAL LIAISON

Characteristics

An individual trained in first aid or trained professionally (LVN, RN, PHN, MD, or paramedic) who can be available at any time during the school day in case of an emergency.

Primary Prevention Activities

1. Educate or encourage the education of a number of individuals in the school to take basic first aid courses.
2. Understand where the nearest emergency rooms are and how best to access them for small and large numbers of injured individuals. Obtain telephone numbers and names of contact people who need to be organized and ready.
3. Develop a list of resource individuals who are knowledgeable and can be relied on to come to the scene of a medical emergency and help with the organization of students as well as help those with minor problems.
4. Develop a plan to get seriously injured persons to the nearest doctor or hospital and also a plan to determine systematically who is in most immediate need of services (triage) in a group of people.
5. Develop procedures to notify the parents of the student in a prompt, tactful, and caring manner.

Secondary Prevention Activities

1. Administer first aid to injured students.
2. Triage injured students and staff. Determine where each should go for services and contact resources (ambulances, parents, etc.) necessary for transportation.
3. Keep a written record of who has received which services and who has been transported where.

Tertiary Prevention Activities

1. Provide ongoing medical and emotional assistance to the ill or injured.
2. Serve as a liaison between the school and hospitalized or home-bound students.

LAW ENFORCEMENT LIAISON

Characteristics

An individual with knowledge of school administrative policies and some understanding of law enforcement.

Primary Prevention Activities

1. Be very clear what constitutes a criminal violation and what constitutes a school disciplinary problem.
2. At what point and in which kinds of crises should police be called immediately.
3. Develop a relationship among administrators, building personnel, and students with the local police authorities.
4. Educate administrators and, if necessary, teachers regarding the policies and standard operating procedures of the local police, including what information is important to collect in order to support law enforcement efforts.

Secondary Prevention Activities

1. Understand under what conditions police can be summoned for help with (a) drug trafficking on campus, (b) violence on campus, (c) suicide threats (on campus or called in), and (d) threats to administrators.
2. Understand the steps and necessary elements involved in involuntary hospitalization and obtaining a mental illness warrant.

Tertiary Prevention Activities

1. Coordinate the reentry to school of students who have been incarcerated or expelled.
2. Coordinate communication between the school system and the juvenile justice personnel such as probation officers.

APPENDIX B

Agency Assistance in Disasters
or Building Crises*

SERVICES FOR CHILDREN

Knowing what kind of assistance is available in the community through government, religious, and private agencies is necessary when responding to the needs of children and families in disasters. There are few federal or state agencies that provide direct services for emotional problems of children. Most services are found in local government and private agencies. Disaster workers need to learn about all the community mental health resources specifically offering services to children and families. Sources of such information are state departments of mental health and members of the professional mental health community.

Some of the probable resources include:

- Community mental health centers.
- County/city mental health departments.
- Family service agencies.
- Public and private child mental health and child guidance agencies.
- Children's hospitals.
- Institutions for exceptional children (schools, residences).
- Professionals in child mental health.

GENERAL ASSISTANCE

The following partial list of agencies available for assistances is taken from the *Training Manual for Human Service Workers in Major Disasters* (Farberow & Fred-

*From Farberow and Gordon (1981).

erick, 1978c) and is included for the convenience of the reader. The services offered are general and cover a wide range of problem areas.

Federal

- *Department of Health and Human Services (HHS).* Public health and welfare functions.
- *Federal Emergency Management Agency (FEMA).* Coordinates all federal services in presidentially declared disasters. It funds the following disaster programs: temporary housing, disaster unemployment assistance, individual and family grants, legal services, and crisis counseling and training. It makes flood insurance available. With the states, FEMA sets up disaster assistance centers.
- *Department of Labor.* Disaster unemployment assistance.
- *Department of Agriculture.* Farmers Home Administration (FHA) disaster loans, food stamps, and food commodities.
- *Small Business Administration.* Disaster loan program for homes and businesses.

State

- *Department of Vocational Rehabilitation.* Medical care and retraining for injured persons.
- *Department of Public Assistance.* Assistance to welfare clients (Federal Assistance Program).
- *Department of Health.* Immunization and preventive health measures as necessary.
- *Department of Mental Health.* Referral for disaster victims with mental health needs.
- *National Guard.* Except when called into federal service.
- *Civil Defense.* Assistance to communities for damage to public facilities; some states have a separate disaster preparedness agency.

Local City/County Government

- The local/county level counterparts of state government provide the following services:
- *City/County Government.* Declaration by public proclamation of emergency when situation cannot be handled by existing relief agencies, private and governmental, operating in the normal manner.
- *Civil Defense.* "Preparation of comprehensive plans and programs for the civil defense in both enemy-caused and natural emergencies."
- *Police Department.* Suppression of criminal activity, dispersal of crowds, traffic control, organization and control within the damaged area, and alerting through telegraph section.

● *Fire Department.* Alerting through telegraph section, minimizing or preventing the effects of fire, assisting with water supply, street clearance, and demolition.

● *Associated General Contractors.* Rescue and engineering services, clearing of streets, repairing of bridges, and bulldozing operations.

● *Department of Health and Hospitals.* Medical services including emergency first aid, ambulance service, etc.

● *Health Division.* Sanitation, immunization, vital statistics, and public health nursing.

● *Coroner's Office.* Collection, identification, and burial of the dead.

● *Department of Streets.* Clearance and maintenance of the streets for traffic, formulating and enforcing emergency traffic regulations in cooperation with police, and garbage/rubbish collection and disposal.

● *Department of Public Utilities.* Rehabilitation and maintenance of water supply, lighting, heating, and power, and coordination of activities by privately owned utilities.

● *Bistate Transit.* Vehicles, fuel, etc.; drivers.

● *Civil Air Control.* Reconaissance and movement of key personnel and light equipment.

● *Telephone Company.* Communications.

● *Radio Amateur Civil Emergency Services (RACES).* Shortwave radio.

● *Radio/TV Networks.* Communications.

● *Human Relations Commission.* Volunteer committee responsible for protection of innocent citizens; subcommittee includes churches.

● *Department of Welfare.* Responsible for all emergency welfare services, including feeding, housing, and financial assistance; augmented by ARC and private social welfare agencies.

Voluntary Agencies

● *American National Red Cross.* In addition to immediate assistance, food, clothing, rent, transportation, temporary home repairs, medical and health needs, selected furnishings and personal occupational supplies, and equipment and other essentials; referring families to government disaster programs, providing additional assistance with major needs to families for whom such government programs are not available.

● *Catholic Charities.* Wide variety of services; differs from one diocese to another.

● *Christian Reform World Relief Committee.* Building advisors, builders, interviewers.

● *Church of the Brethren.* Cleanup, building.

● *Mennonite Disaster Service.* Cleanup, building, some feeding and child care.

● *Salvation Army.* Feeding, shelters, counseling, household furniture, etc.

- *Seventh Day Adventists.* New and used bedding, clothing and comfort kits, diapers (warehousing—Lansing, Michigan).
- *Society of St. Vincent de Paul.* Food, clothing, assistance to aged and infirm, poor, and children.
- *Volunteers of America.* Feeding, sheltering; differs from place to place.
- *Church of the Latter Day Saints (Mormon).* Food, clothing, cleanup, rebuilding, household furniture, mental health counseling.

APPENDIX C

Essential Concepts in the Training
of Crisis Workers*

KNOWLEDGE

1. Crisis theory and principles of crisis management
   a. Origins and development of crisis.
   b. Manifestations of crisis—emotional, cognitive, behavioral, and bio-physical.
   c. Duration and outcomes of crisis, including effective and ineffective crisis coping.
   d. Steps of the crisis management process—assessment, planning, implementation, and evaluation.
   e. Application of the crisis management process to special groups at risk for crisis—drug abusers, victims of abuse, and the chronically mentally ill.
2. Suicidology, including principles of lethality assessment.
3. Victimology, including assessment of assault potential and victimization.
4. Death, dying, and grief work.
5. Principles of communication.
6. Ethical and legal issues regarding suicide, crime, and victimization.
7. Voluntary and involuntary hospitalization criteria.
8. Identification and use of community resources in crisis work.
9. Team relationships in crisis work.
10. The consultation process and its place in crisis management.
11. Principles and structures for record keeping.

*Reprinted with permission from Hoff and Miller (1987).

206

ATTITUDES

1. Acceptance of and nonjudgmental response to persons different from self and toward controversial issues, for example, not discussing the moral rightness or wrongness of suicide or abortion with a person.
2. Balanced, realistic attitude toward oneself in the helper role, for example, not expecting to "rescue" or "save" all potentially suicidal people or to solve all the problems of the distressed person, not expecting a battered woman to leave her abusing husband in spite of the fact that she may be unready because of obstacles she cannot overcome.
3. A realistic and humane approach to death, dying, self-destructive behavior, victimization, and other human issues, including not asking questions of a battered victim such as "What did you do to provoke the beating?" or not implying that a rape victim is at fault for having hitchhiked.
4. Dealing with emotionally laden issues such as AIDS.
5. Coming to terms with one's own feelings about death, dying, and potential for violence, insofar as these feelings might deter one from helping others.

SKILLS

1. Applying the techniques of formal crisis management—assessment, planning, implementation, evaluation (including assessment of victimization and risk of suicide and/or violence toward others).
2. Communicating—listen actively, question discreetly, respond empathetically, and advise and direct appropriately.
3. Mobilizing community resources efficiently and effectively, for example, engaging the rescue squad within 15 minutes of receiving a suicide attempt call, collaborating with the police in a violent situation without escalating the crisis and precipitating more violence, and making an appropriate referral for follow-up counseling or therapy.
4. Implementing policy and keeping records accurately and efficiently, that is, recording essential notes in succinct form within the same work shift so that they are useful to the next crisis worker.
5. Implementing the procedures for voluntary and involuntary hospitalization when indicated.
6. Using the consultative process, that is, knowing whom to call under what circumstances and, in fact, *doing* it.
7. Carrying out these crisis management steps while withholding judgment on controversial behaviors and not imposing values on the person in crisis and his or her family.

APPENDIX D

Materials for Training
of the Paraprofessional Staff*

KEY CONCEPTS

The Target Population Is Primarily Normal

The recipients of help are generally adequate individuals temporarily disrupted by a severe stress but usually capable of functioning adequately under normal circumstances. True, there may be some people who were emotionally disturbed before the crisis and for whom the present upheaval may precipitate a mental illness. However, the task will not be to treat severely disturbed individuals directly but to recognize their needs and to help them receive professional care.

Most of the work at first will be to give more concrete types of help to normal people under stress. Such help includes dispensing information about available services, how to get insurance benefits or loans, assistance with applications at government agencies, health care, baby sitting, transportation, etc. Some of the most important help may be in simply listening, providing a ready ear, and indicating interest and concern.

People do not generally disintegrate in a disaster. Usually they are found pitching in and helping others. However, as frustrations and disillusionment accumulate, more severe emotional reactions may surface.

People respond to active interest and concern. People undergoing great stress and pressure often tend to feel isolated, as if they are alone with their problems. By expressing interest in them and their concerns, by actively involving oneself in their resolution, one provides an invaluable service and usually forestalls much more severe subsequent emotional distress.

People may reject help because of pride. They may feel disgraced because help was

*From Farberow and Frederick (1978a).

needed, or they might not want any help from outsiders. Tact and sensitivity are needed in bringing a new program of assistance into a community. That is why it is best to use as helpers community members who will be seen as neighbors and not as strangers.

Avoid Mental Health Labels

Many people still tend to think of mental health as implying "crazy" or "freakish." Some will refuse if the help is identified in any way as mental health. New terms should be used, such as "human services," "recovery assistance," and "problem resolution."

Be Innovative in Offering Help

Avoid the traditional model. "Human services workers" must be prepared to work in all sorts of situations and under all sorts of conditions. Don't wait for the client to seek help; instead, go out and find her or him. This may be done in outreach or case-finding activities involving leaving the office and knocking on doors or ringing doorbells.

Fit the Program into the Community

Needs will change over time, and they will be different in different areas for many reasons. Subcultures will require special attention in order to meet what may be unique demands, determined by language, ethnicity, etc. The different stages of disaster will present different problems.

ETHICS OF INTERVIEWING—CONFIDENTIALITY AND PRIVACY

A helping person is in a privileged position. Helping someone in need implies a sharing of problems, concerns, and anxieties—sometimes with intimate details. This special sharing cannot be done without a sense of trust, which is built on mutual respect and includes the explicit understanding that all discussions are confidential and private. No cases should be discussed elsewhere without the consent of the person being helped (except in extreme emergency, where it is judged that the person will harm himself or others). It is only by maintaining the trust and respect of the client that the privilege of helping can continue to be exercised.

PROCEDURES FOR HELPING

The basic theory underlying the process of helping is crisis intervention. This theory generally assumes that most people can take care of many problems in their lives. However, when equilibrium is upset by some stress, any person may temporarily be pushed off balance emotionally and show signs of disturbance. He will apply his usual coping mechanisms until he succeeds and the distress subsides. When the emergency is unique and the strain severe, he may not have any effective coping mechanism immediately available, so the person remains highly disturbed. Help is needed, and the help is most useful if provided as soon as possible.

APPENDIX E
Materials for Crisis Drills

MOCK CRISIS

On Wednesday, March 8, at 10:30 A.M., several second-grade girls ran from the girls' restroom yelling "Mrs. Chandler is hurt, Mrs. Chandler is hurt." (Mrs. Chandler is a second-grade teacher.) The nearby first-grade students overheard the frantic cries. Among these students was Ursula Chandler, Mrs. Chandler's first-grade daughter. A second-grade teacher went to the restoom and found Mrs. Chandler lying on the floor. Blood was coming from her head. She was not moving. The teacher quickly notified the nurse to come to the scene.

The children near the restroom were alarmed and crying. Students and staff all over the building were quickly becoming aware that something was wrong.

CRISES INTERVENTION TEAM

Crisis Coordinator/Media Coordinator _____

Counseling/Psychologist Liaison _____

Student Liaison _____

Parent Liaison _____

Campus Personnel Liaison _____

Medical Liaison _____

Law Enforcement Officer/District Communication _____

Crisis Coordinator

As the *crisis coordinator,* what is your response to this crisis?

211

- Call crisis team together and assess situation and clarify various duties.
- Get immediate feedback from nurse's assistant on severity of injury.
- Direct law enforcement liaison to contact superintendent and others regarding situation; also direct designee to follow up as necessary with calls.
- Direct any media representatives to music room and meet with them regarding the situation (would probably not be any for this crisis).
- Work with personnel, parent, and student liaisons to coordinate communication to those groups.
- Hold faculty meeting for debriefing at end of day.
- Meet with crisis team to review actions and improve on our response.

Student Liaison

As the *student liaison*, what is your response to this crisis?

- Ask all students to return to their area and stay with their teachers.
- Ask personnel to move children near restrooms to the cafeteria so emergency medical aid can be easily accessed.
- Work with crisis coordinator to decide on what information would be given to students and by whom.
- Ask counselor to work with injured teacher's daughter.
- Coordinate with the counselor and follow up work with distressed students.

Personnel Liaison

As the *personnel liaison*, what is your response to this crisis?

- Communicate with the staff by memo what has occurred and what needs to be communicated to students at this time. (Coordinate with student liaison.)
- Direct personnel to or from any specific area of the building that would be affected (music room, cafeteria).
- Give updated memo to staff as information becomes available.
- Work with school counselor to meet support needs of staff.
- Help organize and hold debriefing session with staff after school that day.

Parent Liaison

As the *parent liaison*, what is your response to this crisis?

- Contact husband of the injured teacher with available details and plans (nature of injury, hospital?).
- Communicate with parent volunteers in building about nature of incident,

how it is being handled, and how they could help (meet concerned parents at door).

- Direct incoming parent calls regarding incident to designated person who is providing information and reassuring parents that everything is being handled well.
- Direct written communication to all parents (at end of day) about the incident, how it was handled, and the fact that they can call if they have any question or need help.
- Be available for parent follow-up.

Counseling Liaison

As the *counseling liaison*, what is your response to this crisis?

- Give immediate attention to injured teacher's daughter.
- Coordinate with student liaison to meet counseling needs of distressed students (especially those who discovered the injured teacher—immediate counseling and long-term).
- Work with the husband of the victim if necessary.
- Be available to any distressed faculty members or parents.

Law Enforcement Liaison

As the *law enforcement liaison*, what is your response to this crisis?

- Use the hotline to call Superintendent, Public Information Director, Security Director, and Sheriff's Department.
- Direct the medical emergency vehicle to the correct location.
- If the Sheriff's department arrives, answer any questions they may have.

Medical Liaison

As the *medical liaison*, what is your response to this crisis?

- Give immediate first aid to the victim.
- Assess medical emergency and decide if additional medical personnel/EMT is needed.
- If so, direct the crisis assistant to call 911 and give the appropriate information.
- Stay with victim until the EMT arrives.
- If her husband has not arrived, go with victim to the emergency room.
- Follow up with staff members on any outcome of injury.

CRISIS PLAN WORK SHEET

Describe current options used by them _____

_____

_____

List resources available to team _____

_____

_____

List personnel resources available to team _____

_____

_____

Develop Crisis Plan A (run away) _____

_____

_____

Develop Crisis Plan B (temper tantrum) _____

_____

_____

Develop Crisis Plan C (injured child) _____

_____

_____

_____

Describe areas on which team needs to focus to deal with crisis _____

_____

_____

_____

APPENDIX F

Resources for Dealing with Death

Buscaglia, L. (1982). *The fall of Freddie the leaf.* New York: Holt Rinehart & Winston. A thought-provoking view of the balance between life and death through the eyes of a leaf.

Cardy, A. F. (1984). *Dusty was my friend.* New York: Human Sciences Press. An 8-year-old boy proceeds through the stages of the grief process following the death of his friend Dusty in a car accident.

Hammond, J. (1981). *When my dad died.* Ann Arbor: Cranbrook. A child's father dies, and the death is seen through the eyes of the child as the loss is experienced.

Hazen, B. S. (1985). *Why did Grandpa die.* Racine: Western. Molly was very attached to her grandfather, who became ill and died. Molly learns to cope with her feelings of sadness and learns to understand death. Fond memories of her grandfather are carried with her to adulthood.

Krementz, J. (1982). *How it feels when a parent dies.* New York: Knopf. The author conducted interviews with 18 children who experienced the loss of a parent. The children ranged in age from 7 to 16.

LeShan, E. (1976). *Learning to say good-by.* New York: Avon. The stages of mourning are discussed in straightforward terms that a child can understand.

Sanford, D. (1986). *It must hurt a lot: A child's book about death.* Portland: Multnomah. This book details the feelings that a child has when his puppy is killed. The child learns that loss hurts and that other people want to help with grief.

Schaefer, D., & Lyons, C. (1986). *How do we tell the children?* New York: New Market. A step-by-step guide to talking about death with children across developmental stages. Many practical examples are provided.

Viorst, J. (1971). *The tenth good thing about Barney.* Hartford: Atheneum. Barney was the family cat who died. The book describes how a young boy copes with the loss and remembers good things about Barney.

215

APPENDIX G

Crisis Intervention Test

1. Crisis intervention recommendations from the N.I.M.H. include which of the following?
   a. Remember children are resilient.
   b. Mental health workers should seek out those who need help.
   c. Work with the child and the child's parents.
   d. All of the above.

2. Children's reactions to a disaster might include which of the following?
   a. Fear of future disasters.
   b. Loss of interest in school.
   c. Regressive behavior.
   d. Sleep disturbances.
   e. All of the above.

3. Parents can help their child through a crisis by
   a. Being patient and tolerant.
   b. Relaxing behavioral expectations for a short time.
   c. Providing structure.
   d. Rehearsing safety measures to manage a future crisis.
   e. All of the above.

4. The most common reaction by a school to a crisis is which of the following?
   a. Ignore it.
   b. Respond spontaneously.
   c. Respond based on prior planning.

5. It is estimated that ____% of the people who experience a crisis never resolve it.
   a. 25%.
   b. 5%.

    c. 1%.

    d.15%.

6. Public relations is very important following a crisis. The Exxon response to the Valdez oil spill illustrates failure to follow which of the principles?
   a. Mobilize quickly and show concern.
   b. Involve the top executive.
   c. Both a and b.

7. Key strategies to improve school safety advocated by school superintendents from the 15 largest school systems are which of the following?
   a. Involve the public.
   b. Improve school leadership.
   c. Keep guns off campus and halt gang activity.
   d. All of the above.

8. Lessons learned from severe crisis situations at school (i.e., Stockton, Winnetka, Cokeville) were which of the following?
   a. No two crises are exactly alike.
   b. Review crisis policies annually.
   c. A team approach with a clear chain of command is needed.
   d. Schools need a good communication system.
   e. All of the above.

9. The biggest mistake that school employees make when breaking up a fight between students is
   a. They rush in without analyzing the situation and announcing their presence.
   b. They call the students by name.
   c. They disperse the audience.
   d. They give the students choices and refrain from threatening the students involved with consequences.

10. The Right to Safe Schools constitutional amendment is in effect in which state?
    a. Texas.
    b. Montana.
    c. New York.
    d. California.

11. Goals for crisis intervention are which of the following?
    a. Identify the primary problem.
    b. Vent strong emotions.
    c. Set limits and provide referral information.
    d. Provide support and problem-solving assistance.
    e. All of the above.

12. Measures that have been tried at school to improve safety have been which of the following?
    a. Lock all but one door.
    b. Close off stairwells.
    c. Remove faculty restrooms.
    d. Decrease parent access.
    e. All of the above.

13. School administrators downplay crime incidents because
    a. They fear criticism.
    b. They prefer to rely on their own security and discipline system.
    c. They wish to avoid litigation and publicity.
    d. All of the above.

14. Perhaps the best piece of advice in handling a potential crisis at school is
    a. Don't be caught with your plans down.
    b. Get the facts and act quickly to dispel rumors.
    c. Wait a day because the crisis will resolve itself.
    d. It is best to underreact at first.
    e. Both a and b.

15. Disturbed adults report that they attacked the school because of
    a. Negative school memories.
    b. Children are vulnerable.
    c. National publicity for their actions.
    d. All of the above.

16. Various surveys and estimates of weapons and students have found which of the following?
    a. Approximately 100,000 students carry a gun to school every day.
    b. Guns kill 10 children every day.
    c. 41% of boys and 24% of girls report they could get a gun easily.
    d. 23% of boys surveyed said they carried a knife to school at least once last year, and 7% carried a knife daily.
    e. All of the above.

CRISIS INTERVENTION TEST ANSWERS

1. D   All of the above.
2. E   All of the above.
3. E   All of the above.
4. A
5. A
6. C
7. D

8. E
9. A
10. D
11. E
12. E
13. D
14. E
15. D
16. E

APPENDIX H

Sample Crisis Drills

INCIDENT

Secondary

A female student has been shot in the foot by a pistol by the flagpole in front of the school. The pistol, which she was carrying in her purse, discharged with students nearby. Your first notification of the incident is when several hysterical students rush into the office. The student has a younger brother who attends the same school. The superintendent's secretary will role play the mother; please call her.

Elementary

A group of unsupervised boys were playing near a high-voltage tower near the playground. One boy received a severe electrical shock. Your notification of the incident is when several hysterical students rush into the office. It is reported that several students became so frightened that they left the school grounds. The injured boy has younger siblings at the school and an older brother in junior high school. Superintendent's secretary will role play the mother; please notify her.

TASK

The elementary and secondary schools were given their respective scenarios with the following identified task: Please respond to this incident following the district crisis intervention procedures. District personnel are on the scene to role play and ask questions. This is a *practice drill,* and district personnel should be alerted; however it is *not necessary* to notify agencies outside the district.

A crisis visitation team was present to role play the crisis. The team was composed of central administrators. The involvement of top administrators in this activity gave principals the message that it was important. Crisis visitation team members were assigned these specific roles to play:

- Victim
- Bereaved classmate
- Father of the victim
- Law enforcement personnel
- Media representative
- Angry citizen

The crisis visitation team members were given the following directions.

The purpose of the crisis visitation team is to assess the ability of individual schools to respond to a simulated crisis and to give each participating school feedback that will enable them to be better prepared in the event of a real crisis. Administrators in every building have been in-serviced on this topic. Each building has a designated crisis team with the following liaisons: medical, campus, law enforcement, student, parent, and counseling.

Each of you has a designated role in the simulated crisis. Please familiarize yourself with your role and feel free to ask additional questions besides those listed. We are hoping to see evidence of teamwork, prior planning, and anticipation of the ramifications of such a crisis. Please make notes and include your observations of the crisis team's response.

Bereaved Classmate

1. Who is available to comfort you?
2. You are unsure whether to remain at school or go home.
3. Will the school be safe and normal tomorrow?
4. You have other friends who are upset. Who could talk to your friends or to your class?
5. Is your friend going to be all right?
6. How can you help your friend?
7. How could this have happened?

Father of the Victim

1. How were you contacted?
2. What support was offered you and your family?
3. Did school personnel offer to accompany you to the hospital?
4. What follow-up assistance was offered?

Law Enforcement Personnel

1. Who meets you and gives you details of the incident?
2. Will a report be filed on the incident?
3. Who will file the report?
4. Are you allowed to interview witnesses?
5. Are you directed to the hospital to see the victim?
6. Are there additional things to be done to secure the scene?

Angry Citizen

1. How did school personnel interact with you?
2. What plans were stated to make school a safer place?
3. Did school personnel treat you with respect?
4. Did school personnel make note of your suggestions to make school safer?

Victim

1. Who was sent to the scene?
2. How were the nurse and emergency medical team notified?
   a. Was the nurse in the building?
   b. If not, who was called?
   c. What plans were stated to call an ambulance? By whom? Who would meet the ambulance?
   d. What medical assistance would be provided?

The deputy superintendent accompanied the crisis visitation team. He delivered the notification of the crisis by presenting a note to the secretary of the school. The following questions were answered to document the response of the school:

1. Who was identified to go to the scene? Was this a reasonable choice of personnel?
2. Was the building crisis team called in?
3. Were the office of the Superintendent and Public Information Director notified? If so, by whom?
4. What plans were stated to restore order and direct students? By whom?
5. What plans were stated to contact the parents of the injured? By whom?
6. What plans were stated to call the local police? By whom? What plans were stated to call the Director of Security? By whom?
7. What plans were stated to notify the sibling? By whom?
8. What plans were stated to communicate to the faculty what happened? By whom?

9. What plans were made to follow up the medical condition of the injured student? By whom?
10. What plans were made to provide follow-up at school for those most affected? By whom?
11. Was the entire crisis team involved in handling the incident?
12. Was there an emphasis on teamwork?
13. Was it evident that the crisis team had given prior thought to their respective duties?

APPENDIX I

Coordination of District Crisis Intervention Program with Transportation Emergency Procedures

1. Provide psychological first aide at the accident scene. For example:

    Assistance to the Injured

    - emergency first aide should be started
    - do not move the injured
    - reassure the injured, keeping them still and quiet
    - stay with the injured until medical assistance arrives

    Psychological First Aid

    - assure students of their safety and that help is on the way
    - give clear and calm directions to students about what to do, where to go and how they can help
    - understand that normal reactions are anxiety, shock, dismay and some denial
    - minimize undue blaming of others
    - attend to student's feelings but try to reduce negative outbursts by supporting and complimenting those students that are handling the crisis well and following your instructions.

2. The dispatcher plays an important role in your procedures and should call the schools involved and activate the building crisis team. A call to psychological services may also help facilitate activation of the building crisis team.

3. Activities for building crisis team
    A. Initiate immediate communication with superintendent's office, public information director and transportation director and maintain for duration of crisis.

B. Care of students and family at hospital
   1. Team members can support and comfort children and families at the hospital.
   2. Avoid discussion of responsibility of the accident but instead focus on current emotional needs of students and families.
   3. Serve as a communication link between the hospital and the school.
   4. Identify yourselves to emergency personnel.
   5. Ask for aide from chaplain if needed.
C. Dissemination of information at school
   1. Notification with parent permission to the siblings of the injured. Provide support to the siblings until parent arrives. Follow-up to emotional needs of siblings depending on severity.
   2. Precise and accurate information of what has happened should be provided to faculty and students as soon as possible. This will dispel rumors. Emotional support needs to be provided to faculty and students. Students need to be given permission for a range of emotions and an opportunity to express them.
   3. Follow-up at school
      a. classroom discussions need to be provided to allow children to process feelings
      b. the length of time to return to normalcy will vary depending on severity of the crisis and the individual make-up of students
      c. previous losses or tragedies that are unresolved may resurface for students and faculty
      d. students who were hospitalized will need supportive help upon return to school
      e. the building crisis team and transportation personnel need to review the intervention and discuss ways to improve responses in the future.

References

Aguilera, D. C., & Messick, J. M. (1974). *Crisis intervention: Theory and methodology.* St. Louis: C. V. Mosby.

Aharnstam, S., & Woolf, O. (1975). [Kiryat-Shmona Project.] *Havat Daat, 5,* 14–18.

American Association of Suicidology. (1976a). *Standards for administrative structure. Evaluation criteria for the certification of suicide prevention and crisis intervention programs.* American Association of Suicidology, Denver.

American Association of Suicidology. (1976b). *Training procedures. Evaluation criteria for the certification of suicide prevention and crisis intervention programs.* American Association of Suicidology, Denver.

Anderson, L. S. (1976). The mental health center's role in school consultation: Toward a new model. *Community Mental Health Journal, 12,* 83–88.

Andison, F. S. (1977). TV violence and viewer aggression: A cumulation of study results 1956–1976. *Public Opinion Quarterly, 44,* 314–331.

Appleton, W. (1980). The battered woman syndrome. *Annals of Emergency Medicine, 9*(2), 84.

Armstrong, M. (1990a). Emotional reactions to Stockton. In F. Busher (Chair), *Tragedy in Stockton schoolyard.* Symposium presented at the meeting of the National Association of School Psychologists, San Francisco.

Armstrong, M. (1990b). Stockton school shooting. In S. Poland (Chair), *Crises intervention in the schools.* Symposium presented at the meeting of the National Association of School Psychologists, San Francisco.

Auerbach, S. M., & Kilmann, P. R. (1977). Crisis intervention: A review of outcome research. *Psychological Bulletin, 84,* 1189–1217.

Auerbach, S. M., & Spirito, A. (1986). Crisis intervention with children exposed to natural disasters. In S. M. Auerbach & A. L. Stolberg (Eds.), *Crisis intervention with children and families.* Washington, DC: Hemisphere.

Baker, G. W., & Chapman, C. W. (Eds.). (1962). *Man and society in disaster.* New York: Basic Books.

Baldwin, B. A. (1978). A paradigm for the classification of emotional crises: Implications for crisis intervention. *American Journal of Orthopsychiatry, 48,* 538–551.

Baldwin, B. A. (1979). Crisis intervention: An overview of theory and practice. *The Counseling Psychologist, 8,* 43–52.

Banik, S. N. (1984). *Shaping effective mental health services for children and youth.* Washington, DC: Mental Health Services Administration.

Barbanel, L. (1982). Short term dynamic therapies with children. In C. R. Reynolds & T. B. Gutkin (Eds.), *The handbook of school psychology.* New York: John Wiley & Sons.

Bark, E. (1989, April 23). Imagemakers tell clients be honest with the media. *Houston Chronicle,* p. 4e.

Barnes, S. (1989). Psychosocial aspects of wife abuse in the United States. In W. R. Fowler & J. L. Greenstone (Eds.), *Crisis intervention compendium.* Littleton, MA: Copley.

Barrett, T. (1985). *Youth in crisis: Seeking solutions of self-destructive behavior.* Longmont, CO: Sopris West.

Barton, A. (1970). *Communities in disaster: A sociological analysis of collective stress situations.* NY: Doubleday.

Baum, A., Fleming, R., & Davidson, L. M. (1983). Natural disaster and technical catastrope. *Environment and Behavior, 15*(3), 333–354.

Benedek, E. (1979). The child's rights in times of disaster. *Psychiatric Annals, 9*(11), 58–61.

Berger, D. (1989, April 23). Is your child's school bus safe? *Parade Magazine,* pp. 14–15.

Blanford, H., & Levine, J. (1972, July). Crisis intervention in an earthquake. *Social Work, 17,* 16–19.

Blanshan, S. A. (1977). Disaster Body Handling. *Mass Emergencies, 2,* 249–258.

Blanshan, S. A., & Quarantelli, E. L. (1981). From dead body to person: The handling of fatal mass casualties in disasters. *Victomology, 6,* 275–287.

Blauvelt, P. (1990, Fall). School security: Who you gonna call? *National School Safety Center Journal,* pp. 4–8.

Bloom, B. L. (1977). *Community mental health: A general introduction.* Monterey, CA: Brooks/Cole.

Bowers, L. (1989). Follow these guidelines for better and safer playgrounds. *Executive Educator, 11*(4), 27–29.

Bowlby, J. (1960). Separation anxiety. *International Journal of Psychoanalysis, 41,* 89–113.

Boy 9 leads 34 to safety as bus burns. (1987, October 20). *Houston Post,* p. 8a.

Burgess, A., & Holstrom, L. (1974). *Rape: Victims of crisis.* Bowie, MD: Robert J. Brady Co., Prentice-Hall.

Burgess, A., & Holstrom, L. (1980). Sexual trauma of children and adolescents. In L. G. Schultz (Ed.), *The sexual victimology of youth.* Springfield, IL: Charles C. Thomas.

Busher, F. (Chair). (1990). *Tragedy in Stockton schoolyard.* Symposium presented at the meeting of the National Association of School Psychologists, San Francisco.

Butcher, J. N., & Koss, M. P. (1978). Research on brief and crisis oriented psychotherapies. In S. L. Garfield & A. Bergin (Eds.), *Handbook of psychotherapy and behavior change: An empirical analysis* (2nd ed., pp. 725–768). New York: Wiley.

Butcher, J. N., & Maundel, G. R. (1976). Crisis intervention. In I. Weiner (Ed.), *Clinical methods in psychology.* New York: Wiley Interscience.

Canter, L. (1987). *Assertive discipline for bus drivers.* Santa Monica: Canter.

Cantor, D. (1979). Divorce: A view from the children. *Journal of Divorce, 5,* 357–362.

Caplan, G. (1964). *Principles of preventive psychiatry.* New York: Basic Books.

Caplan, G. (1970). *The theory and practice of mental health consultation.* New York: Basic Books.

Caplan, G. (1974). *Support systems and mental health.* New York: Basic Books.

Caplan, G., & Grunebaum, H. (1968, May). Perspectives on primary prevention: A review. *Archives of General Psychiatry, 18,* 555–558.

Carroll, J. L., Harris, J. D., & Bretzing, B. H. (1979). A survey of psychologists serving secondary schools. *Professional Psychology, 10,* 766–770.

Chapman, D. W. (1962). A brief introduction to contemporary disaster research. In G. W. Baker & D. W. Chapman (Eds.), *Man and society in disaster.* New York: Basic Books.

Chodoff, P. (1980). Psychotherapy of the survivor. In J. E. Dimsdale (Ed.), *Survivors, victims, and perpetrators: Essays on the Nazi Holocaust.* New York: Hemisphere.

Clay, V. S. (1976). Children deal with death. *School Counselor, 23,* 175–183.

Clontz, D. (1988, Winter). Juvenile record sharing. *School Safety Journal,* p. 31.

Cobbs, S. (1976). Social support as a moderator of life stress. *Psychosomatic Medicine, 38,* 300–314.

Collison, B. B. (1987). After the shooting stops. *Journal of Counseling and Development, 66*(7), 389–390.

Comstock, G., Chaffee, S., Katzman, N., McCombs, M., & Roberts, D. (1978). *Television and human behavior.* New York: Columbia University Press.

Conoley, J. C., & Conoley, C. W. (1982). *School consultation: A guide to practice and training.* New York: Pergamon Press.

Cook, V. J., & Patterson, J. G. (1977). Psychologists in the schools of Nebraska: Professional function. *Psychology in the Schools, 14,* 371–376.

Cowen, E. L., & Hightower, A. D. (1986). Stressful life events. In S. M. Auerbach & L. Stolberg (Eds.), *Crisis intervention with children and families.* Washington, DC: Hemisphere.

Crabbs, M. (1981). School mental health services following an environmental disaster. *Journal of School Health, 51*(3), 165–167.

Crowe, T. (1990, Fall). Designing safer schools. *National School Safety Center Journal,* pp. 9–13.

Cull, J., & Gill, W. (1982). *Suicide probability scale manual.* Los Angeles: Western Publishing Services.

Cummings, N. A. (1977). Prolonged (ideal) versus short term (realistic) psychotherapy. *Professional Psychology, 8,* 491–501.

Dade teaches kids to say no to guns. (1989, March 19). *Pensacola News Journal,* p. 26a.

Danish, S. J. (1977). Human development and human services: A marriage proposal. In I. Iscoe, B. L. Bloom, & C. C. Spielberger (Eds.), *Community psychology in transition.* New York: Halstead.

Danish, S. J., & D'Augelli, A. R. (1980). Promoting competence and enhancing development through life development intervention. In L. A. Bond & J. Rosen (Eds.), *Competence and coping during adulthood.* Hanover, NH: University Press of New England.

Danzy, E. S. (1989). Crisis intervention: A response to the mental health needs of children and youth. In W. R. Fowler & J. L. Greenstone (Eds.), *Crisis intervention compendium.* Littleton, MA: Copley.

Dillard, H. (1989). Winnetka: One year later. *Communique, 17*(8), 17–20.
Dillard, H. (1990). Crisis in Winnetka. In S. Poland (Chair), *Crises intervention in the schools.* Symposium presented at the meeting of the National Association of School Psychologists, San Francisco.
Dixon, S. L. (1979). *Working with people in crisis.* St. Louis: C. V. Mosby.
Dynes, R. R. (1974). *Organized behavior in disaster* (Monograph No. 3). Newark, DE: Disaster Research Center, University of Delaware.
Dynes, R. R. (1978). Interorganizational relations in communities under stress. In E. L. Quarantelli (Ed.), *Disasters: Theory and research.* Beverly Hills, CA: Sage Press.
Elliot, J. (1989, April 21). Public angry at slow action on oil spill. *U.S.A. Today,* p. 1b.
Ellison, D., & Paasch, H. (1987, October 13). *Houston Post,* p. 1a.
Engel, G. L. (1961). Is grief a disease? A challenge for medical research. *Psychosomatic Medicine, 23,* 18–22.
Erickson, E. (1962). *Childhood and society* (2nd ed.). New York: W. W. Norton.
Erikson, E. H. (1963). *Childhood and society.* New York: W. W. Norton.
Erikson, E. H. (1968). *Identity, youth and crisis.* New York: W. W. Norton.
Farberow, N. C., & Frederick, C. J. (1978a). *Field manual for human service workers in major disasters. DHEW Publication No. (ADM) 78-537.* Rockville, MD: National Institute of Mental Health.
Farberow, N. C., & Frederick, C. J. (1978c). *Training manual for human service workers in major disasters. DHEW Publication No. (ADM) 81-1070.* Rockville, MD: National Institute of Mental Health.
Farberow, N., & Gordon, N. (1981). *Manual for child health workers in major disasters. DHHS Publication No. (ADM) 81-1071.* Washington, DC: U.S. Government Printing Office.
Feder, J. (1989, Spring). Crime's aftermath. *National School Safety Journal,* pp. 26–29.
Finkelhor, D. (1984). *Child sexual abuse: New theory and research.* New York: The Free Press.
Finkelhor, D. (1985). Sexual abuse of boys. In A. Burgess (Ed.), *Rape and sexual assault: A research handbook.* New York: Garland.
Finkelhor, D., & Hotaling, G. (1983). *Sexual abuse in the National Incidence Study of Child Abuse and Neglect (Final report, National Center on Child Abuse, Grant 90-CA840/01).* Durham, NH: Family Violence Research Program, University of New Hampshire.
Fischer, L., & Sorenson, G. (1985). *School law for counselors, psychologists and social workers.* New York: Longman.
Fox, J. A. (1983). *Violence, victimization, and discipline in four Boston public high schools.* Boston, MA: Northeastern University.
Frederick, C. J. (1977). Current thinking about crises or psychological intervention in the United States disasters. *Mass Emergencies, 2,* 43–50.
Freese, A. S. (1984). *Adolescent suicide: Mental health challenge.* New York: Public Affairs Pamphlets.
Friend, T. (1988, December 5). More teens are dying violently. *USA Today,* p. 1d.
Gallessich, J. (1982). *The practice and profession of consultation.* San Francisco: Jossey-Bass.
Gallop, G. (1984). *Youth, alcohol, and drug abuse statistics.* Princeton, NJ: Mimeographed material.
Gallup, G., Jr. (1984). *Youth alcohol and drug abuse statistics.* Mimeographed material, Princeton, New Jersey.

Garmezy, N. (1975). The experimental study of children vulnerable to psychopathology. In A. Davids (Ed.), *Child personality and psychopathology: Current topics (Vol. 2)*. New York: Wiley-Interscience.

Garmezy, N. (1976). *Vulnerable and invulnerable children: Theory, research, and intervention*. Washington, DC: American Psychological Association.

Garmezy, N. (1981). Children under stress: Perspectives on antecedents and correlates of vulnerability and resistance to psychopathology. In A. Rabin, J. Aronoff, A. M. Barclay, & R. A. Zucker (Eds.), *Further explorations in personality*. New York: Wiley Interscience.

Garmezy, N. (1983). Stressors of childhood. In N. Garmezy & M. Rutter (Eds.), *Stress, coping and development in children*. New York: McGraw-Hill.

Garmezy, N., Masten, A., Nordstrom, L., & Ferrarese, M. (1979). The nature of competence in normal and deviant children. In M. W. Kent & J. E. Rolf (Eds.), *The primary prevention of psychopathology, Vol. 3: Social competence in children*. Hanover, NH: University Press of New England.

Garrison, R. (1989, Fall). Gangsters back to the future. *National School Safety Journal*, pp. 20–23.

Gelles, R. J., & Straus, M. A. (1979). Violence in the American family. *Journal of Social Issues, 35,* 15–39.

Georgia Task Force on Alcohol, Marijuana and Other Drugs. 1987. *State survey report*, Atlanta.

Germain, R. B., Brassard, M. R., & Hart, S. N. (1985). Crisis intervention for maltreated children. *School Psychology Review, 14*(3), 291–299.

Giaretto, H. (1981). A comprehensive child sexual abuse treatment program. In P. Mrazek & C. Kempe (Eds.), *Sexually abused children and their families*. Elmsford, NY: Pergamon.

Glasser, W. (1969). *Schools without failure*. New York: Harper & Row.

Glenn, J. (1990, Fall). Training teachers for troubled times. *National School Safety Journal*, pp. 20–22.

Golan, N. (1978). *Treatment in crisis situations*. New York: The Free Press.

Goldsmith, S. (1988, February). Crisis intervention in the schools. *Views, Insights and Perspectives: The Administrators Management Communique, 19*(4), 8–11.

Goldstein, M. (1981). Major factors acting on the early adolescent. In C. D. Moore (Ed.), *Adolescence and stress*. Rockville, MD: National Institute of Mental Health.

Greenstone, J. L., & Leviton, S. C. (1982). *Crisis intervention: A handbook for interveners*. Dubuque, IA: Kendall/Hunt.

Greer, R. (1988, September 30). Shooting suspect kept thinking of own unhappy school days. *Houston Chronicle*, p. 7a.

Guetloe, E. (1988). Suicide and depression: Special education's responsibility. *Teaching Exceptional Children, 20*(4), 24–29.

Guetzloe, . (1988). Suicide and depression: Special education's responsibility. *Teaching Exceptional Children, 20*(4), 24–29.

Guidubaldi, J., Perry, J. D., & Cleminshaw, H. D. (1983). The legacy of parental divorce: A nationwide study of family status and selected mediating variables on children's academic and social competencies. *School Psychology Review, 12,* 300–323.

Hahn, K. (1957). Origins of the Outward Bound Trust. In D. James (Ed.), *Outward bound*. London: Routledge & Kegan Paul.

Haley, J. (1976). *Problem-solving therapy*. San Francisco: Jossey-Bass.

Halpern, H. A. (1973). Crisis theory: A definitional study. *Community Mental Health Journal, 9,* 342–349.

Hansel, N. (1976). *The person in distress.* New York: Human Services Press.

Harkavy-Friedman, J., Asnis, G., Boek, M., & DiFiore, J. (1987). Prevalence of specific suicidal behaviors in a high school sample. *American Journal of Psychiatry, 144,* 1203–1206.

Harper, S. (1989, Fall), AFT safety survey validates problems. *National Safety Journal,* p. 31.

Harris, M., & Crawford, R. (1987). *Youth suicide: The identification of effective concepts and practices in policies and procedures for Texas schools* (Monograph No. 3). Commerce, TX: East Texas State University, Center for Policy Studies and Research.

Hazelwood, H. L. (1986). Crisis in the classroom: Teacher burnout. In W. P. Fowler & J. L. Greenstone (Eds.), *Crisis intervention compendium.* Littleton, MA: Copley Publishing.

Heffron, E. (1975). *Project Outreach final report.* Nanticobe, PA: Hagleton-Nanticobe Mental Health/Mental Retardation Center.

Heller, D. B., & Schneider, C. D. (1978). Interpersonal methods for coping with stress: Helping families of dying children. *Omega, 8,* 319–331.

Herman, J., & Hirschman, L. (1977). Father–daughter incest. *Signs: Journal of Women in Culture and Society, 2,* 735–756.

Hershiser M., & Quarantelli, E. L. (1976). The handling of the dead in a disaster. *Omega, 7,* 195–208.

Hetherington, E. M., Cox, M., & Cox, R. (1977). The aftermath of divorce. In J. H. Stevens, Jr., & M. Matthews (Eds.), *Mother–child, father–child relations.* Washington, DC: National Association for the Education of Young Children.

Hill, R. (1958). Generic features of families under stress. *Social Casework, 39,* 139–150.

Hoff, L. A. (1978). *People in crisis: Understanding and helping.* San Francisco: Addison-Wesley.

Hoff, L. A., & Miller, N. (1987). *Programs for people in crisis: A guide for educators, administrators, and clinical trainers.* Boston, MA: Northeastern University Custom Book Program.

Holmes, T. H., & Rahe, R. H. (1967). The social readjustment rating scale. *Journal of Psychosomatic Research, 11,* 213–218.

Horswell, C. (1991, May 20). Sense of belonging is powerful incentive to join. *Houston Chronicle,* p. 7a.

Inbar, M., & Stoll, C. (1972). *Simulation and gaming in social sciences.* New York: Free Press.

Inwald, R., Brobst, K., & Morrissey, R. (1987). *Hilson adolescent profile manual.* Kew Gardens, NJ: Hilson Research.

Ivey, A. E., & Alschuler, A. S. (1973). An introduction to the field of psychological education. *Personnel and Guidance Journal, 51,* 591–597.

Jacobson, G. F., Strickler, M., & Morely, W. E. (1968). Generic and individual approaches to crisis intervention. *American Journal of Public Health, 58,* 338–343.

Janis, I. L. (1958). *Psychological stress.* New York: John Wiley & Sons.

Jay, B. (1989, January). Managing a crisis in the schools. *National Association of Secondary Schools Bulletin,* pp. 14–17.

Jennings, L. (1989, October 4). Crisis consultants share lessons they learned from school violence. *Education Week,* pp. 1, 27.

Jones, D. (1991, October 29). Educators learn the science of gangs. *USA Today,* p. 8d.

Kaplan, D. M., & Mason, E. A. (1960). Maternal reactions to premature birth viewed as an acute emotional disorder. *American Journal of Psychiatry, 30,* 539–552.

Kathleen Stoneking v. Bradford Area School District, 856-F. 2d 594. (D.C. Cir. 1987).

Kinzie, J. D., Sack W. H., & Angell, R. H. (1986). The psychiatric effects of massive trauma on Cambodian children. *Journal of American Academic Child Psychiatry, 25,* 370–376.

Keen, J. (1989, February 2). USA schools wrestle with kid violence. *USA Today,* p. 1a.

Kell, J. (1990, October 22). F.B.I. says violent crime up 10%. *USA Today,* p. 3a.

Kelly, R., & Berg, S. (1978). Measuring children's relations to divorce. *Journal of Clinical Psychology, 34,* 215–221.

Kendall, P. C., & Braswell, L. (1984). *Cognitive–behavioral therapy for impulsive children.* New York: Guilford Press.

King, M., & Goldman, R. (1988). Crisis intervention and prevention with children of divorce. In J. Sandoval (Ed.), *Crisis counseling, intervention and prevention in the schools.* Hillsdale, NJ: Erlbaum.

Kinzie, J. D., Sack, W. H., & Angell, R. H. (1986). The psychiatric effects of massive trauma on Cambodian children. *Journal of American Academic Child Psychiatry, 25,* 370–376.

Kirn, S. P. (1975, March). *Community mental health centers and disaster: Considerations regarding response during the post-impact period.* Paper presented at the Southeast Psychological Association, Atlanta, Georgia.

Klein, D. C., & Lindemann, E. (1961). Preventive intervention in individual and family crisis situation. In G. Caplan (Ed.), *Prevention of mental disorders in children* (pp. 283–306). New York: Basic Books.

Klingman, , & Eli, (1981). A school community in disaster: Primary and secondary prevention in situational crisis. *Professional Psychology, 12,* 523–533.

Koeppen, A. S. (1974, October). Relaxation training for children. *Elementary School Guidance and Counseling,* pp. 14–21.

Krasner, W., Meyer, L., & Carroll, N. (1977). *Victims of rape (DHEW Publication No. ADM 77-485).* Washington, DC: U.S. Government Printing Office.

Kurdek, L. A., & Siesky, A. E. (1980a). Children's perceptions of their parents' divorce. *Journal of Divorce, 3,* 339–378.

Kurdek, L. A., & Sieksy, A. E. (1980b). The effects of divorce on children: The relationship between parent and child perspectives. *Journal of Divorce, 4,* 85–99.

Lacayo, N., Sherwood, G., & Morris, J. (1981). Daily activities of school psychologists: A national survey. *Psychology in the Schools, 18,* 184–190.

Landis, J. (1956). Experiences of 500 children with adult sexual deviation. *Psychiatric Quarterly Supplement, 30,* 91–109.

Lazarus, R. S. (1980). The stress and coping paradigm. In L. A. Bond & R. C. Rosen (Eds.), *Competence and coping during adulthood.* Hanover, NH: University Press of New England.

Leder, M. (1987). *Dead serious: A book for teenagers about teenage suicide.* New York: Atheneum.

Leviton, S. C., & Greenstone, J. L. (1989). Intervention procedure. In W. R. Fowler & J. L. Greenstone (Eds.), *Crisis intervention compendium.* Littleton, MA: Copley Publishing Group.

Leviton, S. C., & Greenstone, J. L. (1989). A Key to Successful crisis intervention.

In W. P. Fowler & J. L. Greenstone (Eds.), *Crisis intervention compendium.* Littleton, MA: Copley Publishing.

Lewis, M., & Sarrel, P. (1969). Some psychological aspects of seduction, incest and rape in childhood. *Journal of American Academy of Child Psychology, 8,* 606–619.

Lewis, M. S., Gotesman, D., & Gutstein, S. (1979). The course and duration of crisis. *Journal of Consulting and Clinical Psychology, 47,* 128–134.

Lidell, H. G., & Scott, R. (1968). *The Greek–English lexicon.* Oxford: Clarendon Press.

Liebert, R. M., Sprafkin, J. N., & Davidson, E. S. (1982). *The early window: Effects of television on children and youth.* New York: Pergamon.

Lifton, R. J., & Olson, E. (1976). The meaning of total disaster. The Buffalo Creek experience. *Psychiatry, 39,* 1–18.

Lindemann, E. (1944). Symptomology and management of acute grief. *American Journal of Psychiatry, 101,* 141–148.

Lipton, H. (1990). Crisis in New York City Schools. In S. Poland (Chair), *Crisis Intervention in the schools.* Symposium presented at the meeting of the National Association of School Psychologists, San Francisco.

Luepnitz, D. A. (1979). Which aspects of divorce affect children? *Family Coordinator, 1,* 79–85.

Lystad, M. (1985). *Innovations in mental health services to disaster victims.* Rockville, MD: National Institute of Mental Health Center for Mental Health Studies of Emergencies.

Maccoby, J. (1983). The relationship of age to effects of crisis. *Journal of Consulting and Clinical Psychology, 78,* 558–570.

Markley, M. (1991a, October 12). Campus crime prompts vigilance: Parents, students link up for safety. *Houston Chronicle,* p. 30a.

Markley, M. (1991b, October 8). Stiff federal law highlighted to fight guns, drugs in schools. *Houston Chronicle,* p. 15a.

Markley, M. (1991c, September 8). 13 schools seek out weapons with metal detectors. *Houston Chronicle,* p. 16a.

Martin, R. (1989). Physical aggression techniques. In R. Fowler & J. Greenstone (Eds.), *Crisis intervention compendium.* Littleton, MA: Copley Publishing Group.

Mayfield, M. (1986, December 8). Assaults top the list of classroom chaos. *USA Today,* p. 10a.

McBrien, J. (1983). Are you thinking of killing yourself? Confronting students' suicidal thoughts. *The School Counselor, 31*(1), 79–82.

McDermott, J. (1984). *Crime in the school and community. Crime and delinquency.* New York: Sage.

McEvoy, A. (1988a). Shocking violence in schools. *School Intervention Report, 1*(7), 1–3.

McEvoy, A. (1988b). Keeping the school bus safe. *School Intervention Report, 1*(7), 7.

McGee, R. K. (1974). *Crisis intervention in the community.* Baltimore: University Park Press.

McIntyre, M., & Reid, B. (1989). *Obstacles to implementation of crisis intervention programs.* Unpublished manuscript, Chesterfield County Schools, Chesterfield, Virginia.

Meichenbaum, D. (1975). Toward a cognitive theory of self-control. In G. Schwartz & D. Shapiro (Eds.), *Consciousness and self-regulation: Advances in research.* New York: Plenum Press.

Meichenbaum, D. (1977). *Cognitive–behavior modification: An integrative approach.* New York: Plenum Press.

Meichenbaum, D., & Goodman, J. (1971). Training impulsive children to talk to themselves: A means of developing self-control. *Journal of Abnormal Psychology*, 115–126.

Meiselman, K. (1978). *Incest.* San Francisco: Jossey-Bass.

Memmot, C., & Stone, A. (1989, June 15). Firearms and youngsters: Deadly, tragic mix. *USA Today*, p. 3a.

Meyers, J. (1981). Mental health consultation. In T. R. Kratochwill, (Ed.), *Advances in school psychology* (Vol. 1). Hillsdale, NJ: Lawrence Erlbaum.

Miller. W. B. (1975b). *Violence by youth gangs and youth groups as a crime problem in major American cities.* Washington, DC: U.S. Department of Justice, Law Enforcement Assistance Administration, National Institute of Juvenile Justice and Delinquency Prevention.

Modglin, T. (1989, Spring), School crime: Up close and personal. *National School Safety Journal*, p. 9–11.

Moran, K. (1990, September 21). Few attend talk on guns at Ball High. *Houston Chronicle*, p. 4e.

Moran, K. (1991, May 19). Who is a gang member. *Houston Chronicle*, p. 16a.

Morley, W. E., Messick, J. M., & Aguilera, D. C. (1967). Crisis: Paradigms of intervention. *Journal of Psychiatric Nursing*, 5, 537.

Mosher, R. L., & Sprinthall, N. A. (1971). Psychological education means to promote personal development during adolescence. *Counseling Psychology*, 2(4), 3–71.

Moss, C. (1989). Utilizing effective communication skills in crisis intervention. In R. Fowler & J. Greenestone (Eds.), *Crisis intervention compendium.* Littleton, MA: Copley Publishing Group.

Muck, P. (1990, May 21). Gangs they are in the suburbs now. *Houston Chronicle*, p. 1a.

Muir, E. (1988, Fall). The blackboard jungle revisited. *National School Safety Journal*, p. 25–27.

National Crisis Prevention Institute (1986). *Milwaukee: Wisconsin*, 4(3), 85–86.

National Institute of Mental Health. (1975–1984). *Final reports of crisis counseling projects.* Mimeographed materials on file. Rockville, MD: Center for Mental Health Studies of Emergencies.

National School Boards Association. (1984). *Toward better and safer schools: A school leader's guide to delinquency prevention.* Washington, DC: National School Boards Association.

National School Safety Center (1988). *School safety check book.* Malibu, CA: Pepperdine University Press.

National School Safety Center (1989, May). *Drug traffic and abuse in schools* (National School Safety Center resource paper). Malibu, CA: Pepperdine University Press.

National School Safety Center. (1990). *Gangs in schools: Breaking up is hard to do.* Malibu, CA: Pepperdine.

Nelson, E., Slaikeu, K. (1984). *Crisis interventions: A handbook for practice and research* (pp. 247–263). Boston: Allyn and Bacon.

Oates, M. (1988, Fall), Responding to death in the schools. *Texas Association for Counselor Development Journal*, 16(2), 83–96.

Ohio Attorney General. (1979). *The Ohio report on domestic violence.* Columbus, OH: Bureau of Criminal Investigation.

One day in the lives of USA children. (1990, January 8). *USA Today*, p. 1a.

O'Reilley, J. (1983, September 5). Battered wives. *Time*, p. 23.

Peck, M., Farberow, N., & Litman, R. (Eds.). (1985). *Youth suicide*. New York: Springer.

Pedro-Carroll, J. L., & Cowen, E. L. (1985). The children of divorce intervention project: An investigation of a school-based prevention program. *Journal of Consulting and Clinical Psychology, 53*, 603–614.

Perry, H. S., & Perry, S. E. (1959). *The schoolhouse disasters: Family and community as determinants of the child's response to disaster (Disaster Study No. 11, Publication 554)*. Washington, DC: National Academy of Sciences–National Research Council.

Perry, S. E., Silber, E., & Bloch, D. A. (1956). *The child and his family in disaster: A study of the 1953 Vicksburg tornado (Disaster Study No. 5, Publication 394)*. Washington, DC: National Academy of Sciences–National Research Council.

Pfeffer, C. (1986). *The suicidal child*. New York: Guilford Press.

Piller, R. (1990, October 6). In praise of metal detectors. *Houston Chronicle*, p. 29a.

Poland, P. R., & Kirby, M. W. (1976). A model to replace psychiatric hospitalization. *Journal of Nervous and Mental Disease, 162*(1), 13–22.

Poland, S. (1989a). *Suicide intervention in the schools*. New York: Guilford Press.

Poland, S. (1989b). Bus driver inservice. *Communique, 17*(7), 16.

Poland, S. (1990a). Crisis intervention in the schools. *Communique, 18*(5), 21 and 26.

Poland, S. (Chair). (1990b). *Crisis intervention in the schools*. Symposium presented at the meeting of the National Association of School Psychologists, San Francisco.

Poland, S., & Pitcher, G. (1990). Best practices in crisis intervention. In A. Thomas & J. Grimes (Eds.), *Best practices in school psychology* (Vol. 2, pp. 259–275). Washington: National Association of School Psychologists.

Puryear, D. (1979). *Helping people in crisis*. San Francisco: Jossey-Bass.

Rakoff, V., (1966). Children and families of concentration camp survivors. *Canadian Mental Health, 14*, 24–26.

Raphael, B. (1975). Crisis and loss: Counseling following a disaster. *Mental Health in Australia, 1*(4), 118–122.

Rapoport, L. (1962). The state of crisis: Some theoretical considerations. *Social Service Review, 36*(2), 211–217.

Rapoport, R. (1963). Normal crises, family structure, and mental health. *Family Processes, 2*, 68–80.

Rapp, J., Carrington, F., & Nicholson, G. (1987). *School crime and violence: Victims' rights*. Malibu: Pepperdine.

Rappaport, J. (1977). *Community psychology: Values, research and action*. New York: Holt, Rinehart, & Winston.

Redl, F. (1969). Adolescents—just how do they react? In G. Caplan & S. Lebovici (Eds.), *Adolescence: Psychosocial perspectives* (pp. 79–99). New York: Basic Books.

Reiff, R. (1975). Of cabbages and kings. The 1974 Division 27 annual for distinguished contributions to community mental health. *American Journal of Community Psychology, 3*, 185–196.

Reynolds, W. (1987). *Suicidal ideation questionnaire*. Odessa, FL: Psychological Assessment Resources.

Riders and accidents on the USA's school buses. (1989, May 9). *USA Today*, p. 8a.

Ross, C. (1985). Teaching children the facts of life and death: Suicide prevention in the schools. In M. Peck, N. Farberow, & R. Litman (Eds.), *Youth suicide* (pp. 147–169). New York: Springer.

Rota, K. (1989, December 12). Safety changes are still evolving. *USA Today*, p. 1a.

Ruof, S., & Harris, J. (1988). Suicide contagion: Guilt and modeling. *Communique, 16*(17), 8.

Russell, D. (1984). *Sexual exploitation: Rape, child sexual abuse, and workplace harrassment.* Beverly Hills, CA: Sage.

Rutter, M. (1983). Stress, coping and development: Some issues and questions. In N. Garmezy & M. Rutter (Eds.), *Stress, coping and development in children.* New York: McGraw-Hill.

St. John, W. (1986, Fall). How to develop an effective school communication crisis plan. *National Association of Secondary Principals Bulletin*, pp. 21–24.

Sandall, N. (1986). Early intervention is a disaster: The Cokeville hostage/bombing crisis. *Communique, 15*(2), 1–2.

Sandoval, J. (1985). Crisis counseling: Conceptualizations and general principles. *School Psychology Review, 14*(3), 1985.

Sandoval, J. (Ed.). (1985). Mini-series on crisis counseling in the schools. *School Psychology Review, 14*, 255–324.

Sawyer, K. (1985). The right to safe schools. In *National School Safety Center legal anthology* (pp. 114–134). Malibu: Pepperdine.

Schulberg, H. C. (1974). Disaster, crisis theory, and intervention strategies. *Omega, 5*, 77–87.

Schulberg, H. C., & Sheldon, A. (1968). The probability of crisis and strategies for preventive intervention. *Archives of General Psychiatry, 18*, 553–558.

Schulman, N. (1986). A crisis intervention response to the shuttle disaster, *Newslink, 12*(3), 4.

Shootouts in the schools. (1989, November 20). *Time*, p. 116.

Shore, J. H. (1986). Introduction. In J. H. Shore (Ed.), *Disaster stress studies: New methods and findings.* Washington, DC: American Psychiatric Press.

Shore, T, & Vollmer, (1986). Psychiatric reactions to disaster—The Mount St. Helens experience. *American Journal of Psychiatry, 143*(5), 590–595.

Sifneos, P. E. (1960). A concept of emotional crisis. *Mental Hygiene, 44*(2), 169–170.

Signorielli, N., Gross, L., & Morgan, M. (1982). Violence in television programs: Ten years later. In *Television and behavior: Ten years of scientific progress and implications for the 80's.* Washington DC: U.S. Government Printing Office.

Silver, R., Boon, C., & Stones, M. (1983). Searching for meaning in misfortune: Making sense of incest. *Journal of Social Issues, 39*, 81–101.

Slaikeu, K. (1984). *Crisis intervention: A handbook for practice and research.* Boston: Allyn & Bacon.

Slenkovitch, J. (1986, June). School districts can be sued for inadequate suicide prevention programs. *The Schools' Advocate*, pp. 1–3.

Smead, V. (1985). Best practices in crisis intervention. In A. Thomas & J. Grimes (Eds.), *Best practices in school psychology* (pp. 401–415). Kent: National Association of School Psychology.

Smith, K., & Crawford, S. (1986). Suicidal behavior among "normal" high school students. *Suicide and Life Threatening Behavior, 16*, 313–325.

Smith, L. A. (1989). A crisis intervention model. In W. R. Fowler & J. L. Greenstone (Eds.), *Crisis intervention compendium* (pp. 4–12). Littleton, MA: Copley Publishing Group.

Smith, L. L. (1977). Crisis intervention, theory and practice. *Community Mental Health Review, 2*(1), 5–13.

Snider, M. (1990, November 7). Latchkey kids alone with guns. *USA Today,* p. 1d.

Spanier, G., & Castro, R. (1979). Adjustment to separation and divorce: An analysis of fifty case studies. *Journal of Divorce, 2,* 241–253.

Sperling, D. (1990, June 13). U.S. men face the highest murder risk. *USA Today,* p. 1a.

Spirito, A., & Finch, A. (1980). *A stress inoculation manual for anxiety in children.* Unpublished manuscript, Virginia Commonwealth University, Richmond, VA.

Staff. (1988). *School safety checkbook, National School Safety Center.* Malibu: Pepperdine.

Steele, B., & Alexander, H. (1981). Long-term effects of sexual abuse in childhood. In P. Mrazek & C. Kempe (Eds.), *Sexually abused children and their families.* Elmsford, NY: Pergamon.

Stevens, R. (1989, October). *Safety in the schools.* Crisis intervention workshop, Houston, TX.

Stolberg, A. L., & Garrison, K. M. (1985). Evaluating a primary prevention program for children of divorce: The divorce adjustment project. *American Journal of Community Psychology, 13,* 111–124.

Students offer peers safe ride home. (1990, October 3). *Houston Chronicle,* p. 8a.

Stevens, R. (1990, Fall). Don't get caught with your plans down. *National School Safety Journal,* pp. 4–8.

Stevenson, R. (1986, December). How to handle death in the schools. *National Association of Secondary Principals Bulletin,* pp. 1–2.

Stolberg, A. L., & Anker, J. M. (1983). Cognitive and behavioral changes in children resulting from parental divorce and consequent environmental changes. *Journal of Divorce, 7,* 23–41.

Stolberg, A. L., Camplair, C., Currier, K., & Wells, M. (1987). Individual, familial and environmental determinants of children's post-divorce adjustment and maladjustment. *Journal of Divorce,*

Stolberg, A. L., Kiluk, D. J., & Katherine, M. G. (1986). A temporal model of divorce adjustment with implications for primary prevention. In S. M. Auerbach & A. L. Stolberg (Eds.), *Crisis intervention with children and families.* Washington, DC: Hemisphere.

Straus, M. (1981). *Behind closed doors: Violence in the American family.* Garden City, NY: Anchor Books.

Students offer peers safe ride home. (1990, October 9). *Houston Chronicle,* p. 8.

Surgeon General Report. (1971). *Television and growing up: The impact of television violence.* Washington, DC:

Swift, C. (1978). Sexual exploitation of children in the United States. In *Research into violent behavior: Overview and sexual assaults (Hearings before the Subcommittee on Domestic and International Scientific Planning, Analysis and Cooperation of the Committee on Science and Technology, U.S. House of Representatives), No. 64* (pp. 323–366). Washington, DC: U.S. Government Printing Office.

Swift, C. (1986). Community intervention in sexual child abuse. In S. Auerbach & A. Stolberg (Eds.), *Crisis intervention with children and families.* Washington, DC: Hemisphere.

Taplin, J. R. (1971). Crisis theory: Critique and reformulation. *Community Mental Health Journal, 7,* 13–23.

Taylor, V. A., Ross, G. A., & Quarantelli, E. L. (1976). *Delivery of mental health services in disasters: The Xenia tornado and some implications* (Monograph series No. 11). Columbus, OH: Ohio State University, Disaster Research Center.

Taylor, V. A., Ross, G. A., & Quarantelli, E. L. (1976). Delivery of mental health services in disasters: The Xenia tornado and some implications (Monograph No. 11). Newark, DE: Disaster Research Center, University of Delaware.

Teacher's foresight helps class scare off suspect. (1987, October 13). *Houston Post,* p. 1.

Terr, L. C. (1983). Chowchilla revisited: The effects of a psychic trauma four years after a school bus kidnapping. *The American Journal of Psychiatry, 12,* 140.

Texas Education Agency. (1988, June). *Texas Education Agency/Texas Department of Mental Health Mental Retardation.* Texas: Joint Task Force on Emotional Disturbance.

Tierney, K. J., & Baisden, B. (1979). *Crisis intervention programs for disaster victims: A source book and manual for smaller communities. DHEW Publication No. (ADM) 79-675.* Washington, DC: DHEW.

Titchner, J. L., & Kapp, F. T. (1976). Family and character change at Buffalo Creek. *American Journal of Psychiatry, 113,* 295–316.

Toby, J. (1984). Violence in school. In *Crime and justice: An annual review of research.* Institute for Criminological Research, Rutgers University. Washington, DC: National Institute of Mental Health.

Toffler, A. (1971). *Future shock.* New York: Bantam Books.

Tuckman, A. (1973). Disaster and mental health intervention. *Community Mental Health Journal, 9*(2), 151–157.

Turner, B. (1989, Fall). California's safe schools law tested. *National School Safety Journal,* p. 33.

Tyhurst, J. S. (1951). Individual reactions to community disaster. *American Journal of Psychiatry, 107,* 764–769.

Tyhurst, J. S. (1957). *The role of transition states—including disaster—in mental illness.* Paper presented at Symposium on Preventive and Social Psychiatry, Walter Reed Army Institute of Research and the National Research Council, Washington, DC.

University of Michigan Institute for Social Research. (1987). *National Survey of High School Drug Abuse.* Washington, DC: National Institute on Drug Abuse.

U.S. Department of Health and Human Services. (1981). *National study of the incidence and severity of child abuse and neglect: Study findings. (DHHS Publication No. OHDS-81-30325).* Washington DC: U.S. Department of Health and Human Services.

Vidal, J. (1986, October). Establishing a suicidal prevention program. *National Association of Secondary School Principals Bulletin,* pp. 68–72.

Waddell, D., & Thomas, A. (1989). *Children and responses to disaster: Formulating a disaster plan.* Unpublished handout, National Association of School Psychologists, Silver Springs, Maryland.

Waiting period can curb handgun toll. (1990, June 13). *USA Today,* p. 10a.

Wallerstein, J. S. (1983). Children of divorce: The psychological tasks of the child. *American Journal of Orthopsychiatry, 53,* 230–243.

Wallerstein, J. S., & Kelley, J. B. (1980). *Surviving the breakup: How children and parents cope with divorce.* New York: Basic Books.

Walters, F. (1975). *Physical and sexual abuse of children: Causes and treatment.* Bloomington, IN: Indiana University Press.

Weapons in schools (resource paper). (1990). Encino, CA: National School Safety Center.

Werner, J. S., & Smith, V. (1982). Longitudinal studies on the invulnerable child. *Journal of Developmental Psychology, 75,* 414–434.

West, L. J. (1984). *Alcoholism and related problems: Issues for the American Public.* Englewood Cliffs, NJ: Prentice-Hall.

Wilhelm, R. (1967). *The book of changes or the I Ching.* Princeton, NJ: Princeton University Press.

Wilson, P.G.H. (1988). Helping children cope with death. In J. Sandoval (Ed.), *Crisis counseling, intervention, and prevention in the schools.* Hillsdale, NJ: Lawrence Erlbaum.

Wise, P. S., & Smead, V. S. (1989). Establishing the need for crisis intervention in rural schools. In W. R. Fowler & J. L. Greenstone (Eds.), *Crisis intervention compendium.* Littleton, MA: Copley Publishing Group.

Wolf, R. (1991, May). Showdown over gun control. *USA Today,* p. 1a.

Worden, W. J. (1982). *Grief counseling and grief therapy.* New York: Springer.

Worn school bus aides rescue team. (1989, November 19). *Houston Chronicle,* p. 4.

Youngsters learn to settle conflicts without violence. (1991, October 24). *Houston Chronicle,* p. 1d.

Zarle, T. H., Hartsough, D. M., & Ottinger, D. R. (1974). Tornado recovery: The development of a professional–paraprofessional response to a disaster. *Journal of Community Psychology,* 2, 320–331.

Zizzo, F. (1989). A field experience model for crisis intervention. In W. P. Fowler & J. L. Greenstone (Eds.), *Crisis intervention compendium.* Littleton, MA: Copley Publishing.

Index